Misadventures in Health Care

INSIDE STORIES

Misadventures in Health Care

INSIDE STORIES

Edited by

MARILYN SUE BOGNER
Institute for the Study of Human Error, LLC

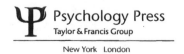

Psychology Press
Taylor & Francis Group

New York London

First Published by Lawrence Erlbaum Associates, Inc., Publishers
10 Industrial Avenue
Mahwah, New Jersey 07430

Reprinted 2008 by Psychology Press

Library of Congress Cataloging-in-Publication Data

Misadventures in health care : inside stories / edited by Marilyn Sue Bogner.
    p.   cm.
   Includes bibliographical references and index.
   ISBN 0–8058–3377–3 (cloth) — ISBN 0–8058–3378–1 (paper)
   1. Medical errors. 2. Primary care (Medicine)—Safety measures. 3. Medical
care—Quality control. 4. Hospital care—Safety measures. 5. Diagnostic errors—
Prevention. 6. Medicine—Practice—Safety measures. I. Bogner, Marilyn Sue.
   R729.8.H857 2003
   610—dc21   2003042849

Printed in the United States of America
10 9 8 7 6 5 4 3 2

*To the professional and lay health care providers
who have prevented untold numbers of adverse outcomes
through their persistent and ingenious efforts
to outwit error-inducing conditions.*

Contents

Series Foreword

Marilyn Sue Bogner

Institute for the Study of Human Error, LLC

Error is ubiquitous—there is no industry, indeed no aspect of life, that is immune to it and its consequences. The desire for safety also is ubiquitous, and the mere mention of error can raise the specter of an unsafe, threatening condition. Error knows no geographical, political, or ideological boundaries. It is a significant real-world problem that needs immediate and concerted attention to reduce its occurrence and enhance safety. This book series brings error and safety to the attention of the global community.

The typical response to an accident in which a person is involved is to say the person was at fault, it was human error; the person committed an unsafe act. There is no denying that the person committed the act; however, the conclusion that the individual was the source of the error most likely is not supported by fact because behavior reflects the interaction of the person and the environment. Nonetheless, remedial activities are directed to the person. Typically, those activities achieve less than the anticipated goal of reducing the likelihood of the error recurring. This book series communicates information about such lessons learned.

Reports of formal investigations of accidents attributed to human error typically are submitted to the source that commissioned, funded, or directed the investigation. Few if any persons except the investigators and members of the supporting organization have access to the reports; hence information from such extended studies is not available to individuals who might incorporate it in their accident prevention and safety promotion activities. Findings from such investigations also can be valuable to students and researchers in determining topics for study and exploration. This book series is the venue for sharing otherwise unavailable information.

There is no academic discipline that is dedicated to the study of error, hence no departments of human error, probably few if any academic courses on error qua error, although the subject may be considered in lectures on topics such as risk, safety, engineering, psychology, and human factors. Because there is no academic discipline focused on human error, there is no driving, coalescing force for sharing knowledge on the topic, no fertile ground for growing human error experts. This book series, by publishing the work of widely dispersed individuals, is a coalescing force, a source for identifying colleagues for collaborative endeavors, and a means for cross-fertilizing ideas.

Work that addresses human error is published in a variety of sources such as proceedings of various professional meetings and chapters in books on assorted topics. This dissipates the information conveyed by those writings when it should be consolidated to build a body of knowledge of human error and safety. This book series develops such a body of knowledge.

This volume, the first in the series, considers human error as a phenomenon to be understood so it can be effectively addressed, thus enhancing safety. This involves challenging the presumption that to err is human and supplanting it with a synthesis of insights conveyed by stories from the rarely considered perspective of health care providers—those who know firsthand what can be involved in an error as well as the myriad of unsafe factors in the context in which health care is provided.

The discussions in this book intentionally are free of the language and constraints of academic disciplines so members of the general population, as well as students of all disciplines, can readily understand the issues and apply them in their personal or professional frame of reference. For the same reason, no solutions are proposed; the readers are free to apply their knowledge and insights to draw their own conclusions.

Foreword

Alphonse Chapanis, Professor Emeritus
Johns Hopkins University

The second half of the 20th century has witnessed advances in medical practice and technology that can only be described as spectacular. The discovery of penicillin in 1928 and its first use to treat wounded soldiers in World War II forecast a dramatic increase in the number of drugs available to the modern practitioner. Not only have new drugs appeared in profusion, but also new methods of manufacturing them—genetic engineering, for example—have been devised. As a result, the U.S. Pharmacopoeia lists thousands of clinically approved drugs worthy of consideration, a number that taxes the capacity of human memories. Although the benefits of these developments cannot be denied, we have also become acutely aware that they have created new problems, because, for one thing, we are continually discovering complex interactions among drugs, and between drugs and the people who take them.

In another arena, artificial hip joints were first implemented in 1928. They, and the first kidney implant in the 1950s and the first heart transplant in 1967, paved the way for the tens of thousands of joint and organ replacements now performed each year. Today's replacements include the hips, knees, shoulders, wrists, heart, lungs, liver, heart valves, kidneys, pancreas, bone marrow, skin, and cornea and lens of the eye. Even as I write, I have read about the first total human hand replacement. Who can foresee what developments will follow that achievement?

Medical technology has more than kept pace with these other advances. Physicians had some specialized machines—for example, electrocardiographs, electroencephalographs, X-ray equipment and renal dialysis machines—prior to 1950, but the years after that saw the development of even more sophisticated and complex equipment—lasers, computerized tomography, magnetic resonance imagery, positron emission tomography, microprocessor-based physiological monitoring systems, mechanical cardiopulmonary bypass systems, and virtual imaging. Personal devices, such as implantable cardiac defibrillators, cochlear implants, and infusion pumps, have also been developed within the past 50 years to increase the quality of daily life for people with certain kinds of defects.

All these advances have been made in a greatly changed and changing environment. People are living longer but at a cost. The emphasis on cost containment by managed care programs has altered the way medical and health services are provided. One consequence is that a substantial amount of health care is now carried out in the home by lay persons who have had marginal, if any, training. These people often have to use and maintain complex medical equipment that was designed to be operated by trained persons. As a result, health care providers sometimes work under conditions that almost literally invite error.

All the advances that have been made in these five decades have had one major drawback: They have increased enormously the opportunities for accidents attributable to human error. Simply stated, there are today vastly increased numbers of ways in which people can make mistakes.

Ask anyone about the causes of everyday errors or accidents and you are almost certain to hear that they are due to such things as carelessness, haste, fatigue, risk-taking, inexperience, or lack of training. In this respect, the convictions of experts, such as designers, engineers, and lawyers, tend not to differ from those of lay people. A common feature of these convictions is that the person committing the error is to blame and that the technology involved is blameless. These attitudes have even pervaded the medical field, as a result of which nurses, physicians, pharmacists, and sometimes medical directors have been forced to suffer reprimands, lose their positions, or even resign.

Meanwhile, at about the same time as all these medical advances were being made, an entirely different technical discipline was born and maturing. This discipline, human factors or ergonomics, largely a product of World War II, looked at errors and accidents in quite a different light. Of course people do things in unintended ways, it acknowledged, everyone does at sometime or another, but to label them human error and to stop at that contributes nothing to their elimination.

In its infancy, this new discipline focused on the displays—the dials, gauges, indicators, printed materials from which people receive information about machine functioning—and on controls—the knobs, levers, cranks, and push buttons people use to direct and issue commands to machines. Through redesign of these devices, human factors found that errors and accidents could, in many instances, be dramatically reduced.

As it matured, human factors broadened its purview and now focuses on all the circumstances in which errors occur—the equipment, environment, procedures, users, skill levels, training, or generically, the system—and asks, "What is there about the system that allows a person to commit an error?" and "How could the system be changed or redesigned so that it would be difficult or impossible for even fallible humans to make mistakes?" In studying systems, this new discipline uses a number of powerful techniques—activity analysis, critical incident study, task analysis, fault tree analysis, failures modes and effects analysis, link analysis—that differ from the controlled experimentation of the laboratory scientist.

When applied systematically this approach has been shown to decrease dramatically errors and accidents in the home, in offices, in factories, on our highways, and in the air. Applications in the medical arena began to appear somewhat later. My 1959 study with Safren[1] was one of the first, if not the first, to use the critical incident technique to study hospital medication errors. Over a period of 7 months we were able to collect 178 error accounts; of those, 143 (80%) were actual errors and 35 (20%) were near errors. Some of them were frightening. For example, in some cases a patient might receive 10 times (or 1/10th), and, in rare instances, 24 times (or 1/24th) the prescribed dosage of a drug. We were able to classify all incidents in seven major types, the three most common ones being that: the wrong patient received a medication, a patient received a wrong dose of medication, or a patient received an extra (unordered) dose of medication. Looked at another way, the three most common immediate causes of the incidents were: failure to follow required checking procedures, misreading or misunderstanding written communications, and transcription errors. More important than the data are the recommendations we were able to make for reducing errors of this kind. They concern virtually every aspect of the medication system: written communication, medication procedures, the working environment, and training and education.

After 1960 the application of the systems approach to medical error began to appear in scattered sources with greater frequency. This book is one of the first to bring this material together and to provide explicit examples of the systems approach to the analysis of errors and accidents in health care. It is an edited collection of 13 chapters written for this book by acknowledged authorities in their respective areas in the United States and abroad. The chapters cover a wide range of health care situations, from emergency rooms and surgeries to homes. They describe adverse outcomes that have occurred in those situations, and the circumstances that led to those outcomes. In so doing, they convey new

---

[1] Safren, M. A., & Chapanis, A. (1959). A critical incident study of hospital medication errors. *Hospitals, May 1,* 16, 1060.

perspectives to our understanding of the factors that contribute to medical error, perspectives that are certain to become more and more critical as medical practice and technology increase in complexity and sophistication.

This book should be widely read not only by researchers and practitioners in all the medical specialties, but also by professionals in the social sciences, human factors, and engineering. Indeed, it should be read by lay persons as well because it contains messages for everyone interested in the integrity of medical care and practice. And who, these days, is not?

Preface:
The Other Perspective

Human error in health care strikes fear in the heart of every person who ever has been, is, or anticipates receiving health care. People trust health care providers with their lives; even the remote possibility of error can be considered a betrayal of that trust. Such trust is necessary for the person seeking treatment for a disorder because what transpires in the process of providing health care, unlike other professional services, is a mystery to the nonprofessional.

People do not know what actually happens when they receive health care. Except for using over-the-counter health care products, few people—even medical device designers who are not health care providers—have experience providing care or using medical devices to treat actual patients in the real world. Even those who are involved in self-care as in managing a chronic disease or providing home care for another individual cannot comprehend what health care professionals do, cannot share their perspective.

Unlike piloting a plane or driving a car, there are no video games to simulate health care. Although health care and the practice of medicine have been the topic of movies and television programs, some of which provide graphic depictions of surgery, they do not provide a vicarious experience of providing care or performing surgery, so people's knowledge of what that entails is vague at best. Because of the lack of health care related experience, the patients and their families are not aware of the conditions that impact the provision of care; they are aware only of their perspective when they receive health care, not of the other perspective—that of the care provider.

People cannot shed light on the mystery of what is involved in the process of providing health care because their experiences when obtaining care—even observing the physical layout of a health care facility—are compromised due to their anxiety about their disorder. When people experience various treatments, diagnostic testing, or surgery their cognitive and observational abilities are affected by illness, medication, pain, or anesthesia. Patients feel they are not in control of the situation, they do not know what is happening, they do not know what the care provider, typically the physician, is doing. Patients can't empathize with the care provider; indeed, they may feel threatened.

Because the process of providing health care essentially is opaque to the patient, when an adverse outcome (side effects, prolonged treatment, injury or death) occurs, even if that outcome is an acknowledged possible consequence of the treatment, people attribute its cause to the only apparent source of the problem—the health care provider. This attitude is apparent not only in people's discussion of how they were wronged by care providers; it also is expressed in numerous books of health care horror stories in which the profound problems the patient suffered are attributed to the care providers.

The patients' and their families' response to a presumed error is anger and the urge for retribution. This anger is heightened by a sense of betrayal; the patients' trust in the care provider was betrayed by the error. The collaborative relationship that should be the essence of health care is corrupted into a counterproductive adversary situation. From the patients' perspective, an error is a willful act by the care provider, either of doing or of *not* doing something, being lax, careless, even negligent—all actions presumed to be totally under the control of the care provider and not influenced by factors other than their motivation. What of the other perspective, that of the care provider?

Typically there is little or no concern about the effect of the error on the care provider. It is common for health care professionals to be trained that they are responsible for whatever happens to their patients, so if an adverse outcome occurs, they may consider themselves accountable—including when the outcome is attributed to error. Care providers tend not to share their perspective with patients; however, sharing that perspective can be useful in addressing the outcome of an error.

When a healthy child who was to undergo elective surgery died as the result of an error, the care provider who was involved with the error explained what happened, gave his perspective, to the grieving parents. Although the parents were distressed by the child's death, they did not express outrage and demand retribution for the error. Rather, they expressed appreciation for being told, were gratified that safeguards were in place to prevent the same error happening again, and did not initiate litigation. This underscores the importance of the perspective of the care provider. Indeed, as that care provider's perspective of the incident gave the parents an understanding of what transpired in the error that killed their child, the perspective of a person who, by being involved in an error, actually experienced its dynamics can contribute significantly to the understanding of human error.

A great deal of research has been conducted, many papers have been written and talks presented about error in health care, but little if any attention has been given to the ultimate authority on error, the experience of the person who allegedly committed it. This book presents such experience through stories relating the perspectives of a variety of health care providers in situations that can and do occur.

Each of the chapters from 2 through 12 presents the perspective of health care providers via stories of episodes of health care in which an error occurred. Following the story, each chapter author identifies and discusses issues related to the error portrayed in the story. By design, no solutions are proposed to address those issues; the stories are case studies to be read for their insights into the causes of error, to be analyzed and possible solutions developed to meet the specific interests and concerns of the reader.

Each story is from the perspective of a different individual care provider— some chapters describe a situation from the perspective of more than one care provider, such as a nurse and a hospital pharmacist. In those stories, each care provider's perspective is addressed independently of the other. This is done to emphasize the fact that every person has their own unique perspective of a situation. The perspectives of more than one person for a given occurrence can be quite different, as is so powerfully portrayed in Kurosawa's 1950 movie *Rashomon* in which eyewitnesses to a murder describe quite different situations.

Each of the stories describes at least one episode of health care during which an adverse event, an error, but not necessarily an adverse outcome of prolonged treatment, injury or death occurred; some chapters present more than one story. The stories describe episodes in a variety of settings in the health care network such as hospitals, physicians' offices, and pharmacies. The order of the chapters (hence, the order of the stories) follows to a degree the progression a person might experience through the various aspects of the health care network should they enter via the emergency room and ultimately be discharged into the community. There is no consistent person throughout the stories. Each story is independent of the others; each has its own cast of characters, which often is integral to the points being made in the chapter. Each chapter can be read independently of the others; however, the messages conveyed in the chapters will be better appreciated if the background for the stories presented by Bogner in chapter 1 is read first.

The vicarious experiences in the world of health care through the perspectives of care providers begins with Linden's consideration of the procedure of transfusing blood in a hospitalized patient (chapter 2)—a ubiquitous occurrence in the emergency department and operating room and to varying degrees elsewhere in a hospital. Mackenzie and Xaio present the perspective of a care provider assisting in a difficult procedure in a shock trauma center (chapter 3). The reader then is provided the perspectives of care providers in an aspect of health care that rarely is observed by a non-health care professional, that of surgery.

In chapter 4, Berguer provides the health care provider's perspective of a traditional open surgical procedure where there is a direct view of the surgical site and the surgeon's hands directly manipulate the organs. The perspectives in the chapter by MacKenzie, Lomax, and Ibottson (chapter 5) and that by Matern (chapter 6) are of care providers performing laparoscopic surgical procedures. Those procedures are conducted using long, thin instruments inserted into the body cavity through small incisions with the surgical site inside the patient being viewed via images from a tiny video camera on a monitor.

In the description of the perspective of a care provider administering anesthesia and the accompanying discussion of the relevant issues (chapter 7), Weinger attests that providing anesthesia is not the simple task a lay person might presume. The care provider's perspective in the chapter by Seagull and Sanderson (chapter 8) raises issues pertaining not only to a pervasive problem in technologically sophisticated health care in the operating room, that of alarms and noise, but also error-related issues for a left-handed care provider. Following surgery under some conditions, the patient is admitted to an intensive care unit (ICU). The perspective of a health care provider in an ICU described by Donchin (chapter 9) points to the rarely considered affects of a health care setting on the health care provider as well as the patient.

After hospital treatment has ended, the next stop in the journey through the health care network for many is home care. Home care, although one of the fastest growing industries in the country, is perhaps the least considered in terms of error and adverse events. The perspective of the care provider in the chapter by Korniewicz and El-Masri (chapter 10) and the discussion of it in that chapter illustrate a number of disquieting issues in home care—issues for the patient and issues for the care provider.

Issues of self-care in the elderly are presented in the story by Park and Skurnik (chapter 11) through the perspective of each member of an elderly couple and that of their daughter as they cope with their medications. These are important perspectives to consider because elderly persons comprise the most rapidly increasing proportion of the population of the United States. The perspectives of health care professionals described by Dandurand (chapter 12) describe a number of error-related issues regarding the settings for dispensing medications, in a hospital pharmacy as well as a community pharmacy, and issues pertaining to the medications themselves. These and other issues from the perspectives in this chapter are pervasive in dispensing the ever-growing number of prescription drugs.

The final chapter of the book (chapter 13) applies lessons learned from industry to the analogy of error as a dramatic performance to identify insights on the causes of error provided by the inside stories of the perspectives of the various health care providers. Bogner proposes an analogy-based template for mining the perspective of the health care provider involved in an error to identify factors that contributed to it. Such knowledge integrated as appropriate with that from the synthesis of knowledge from the perspectives of other health care providers can identify error-inducing factors to be changed to reduce error and adverse outcomes.

ACKNOWLEDGMENTS

The editor of this volume thanks Bill Webber, Anne Duffy, and Debbie Ruel of Lawrence Erlbaum Associates—Bill for his support, helpfulness, enthusiasm, patience and enduring kindness, Anne for her assistance in the early stages of this endeavor, and Debbie for her responsiveness and professionalism. The editor also thanks the chapter authors for their willingness to provide insightful perspectives of very believable care providers—your points certainly are well made. An expression of gratitude also to members of the editor's furry family of two black cats and four deerhounds, who kept constant vigil during her sometimes long and often very late hours at work on this book.

—*Marilyn Sue Bogner*

Contributors

Ramon Berguer, MD, is an associate professor of surgery at the University of California Davis and practices as a general surgeon at the VA Northern California Health Care System and Contra Costa Regional Medical Center in Martinez, California. His research interests include the ergonomic assessment and improvement of the surgical operating room and human factors issues related to human performance and teamwork in surgery. Dr. Berguer is particularly interested in the measurement and interpretation of physical and mental workload in real-work environments. He speaks internationally on these subjects and provides ergonomics consulting services to medical manufacturers.

Marilyn Sue Bogner, PhD, is president and chief scientist of the Institute for the Study of Human Error, LLC, where she serves her clients by identifying system factors that contribute to error. Previously she was employed by U.S. government agencies, addressing the contribution of equipment design to user error, use and error issues in military equipment, and cross-cutting issues in health services. At the Institute of Medicine, National Academy of Sciences, she addressed issues related to quality of primary medical care. In addition, she taught in the psychology and engineering departments at several universities. Dr. Bogner edited and contributed to the book *Human Error in Medicine,* published in 1994 by Lawrence Erlbaum Associates (LEA), and is editor of LEA's book series Human Error and Safety. She is on the editorial board of *Human Factors* and is a reviewer for several professional journals. She has published widely on error and performance issues in book chapters and professional publications and has spoken extensively to professional meetings in the United States and abroad. Dr. Bogner is a Fellow of the American Psychological Association, the Human Factors and Ergonomics Society, and the Washington Academy of Sciences. She holds a BS in mathematics and psychology, and an MA and PhD in psychology.

Alphonse Chapanis, PhD, DSc, received his BA from the University of Connecticut in 1937 and his MA and PhD degrees from Yale in 1942 and 1943, respectively. He was awarded an honorary DSc degree from the University of Connecticut in 1998. He is a Certified Human Factors Professional (CHFP). In 1943 he was commissioned a second lieutenant in the Air Corps, and sent to the School of Aviation Medicine, Randolph Field, Texas, where he was trained as an aviation physiologist. He was then transferred to the Aero Medical Laboratory, Wright Field, Dayton, Ohio, where he conducted research on problems of high-speed, high-altitude flight. He left the Air Force in 1946 with the rank of captain. In 1946 Chapanis joined The Johns Hopkins University and was continuously associated with the university until his retirement in June 1982. He is a professor emeritus from the university. During the academic year 1960–1961, he took a leave of absence to serve as a liaison scientist in the Office of Naval Research Branch Office in the Embassy of the United States, London. Dr. Chapanis is considered a pioneer of the field of human factors. *Applied Experimental Psychology: Human Factors in Engineering Design,* which he co-authored in 1949, was the first textbook in the field. Since then he has published four other books, edited a sixth, and co-authored a seventh. In addition, he has published nearly 200 scientific and professional articles dealing with topics in general experimental psychology, vision, statistics, research design, safety, and human engineering. He has given more than 200 lectures, keynote speeches, and invited addresses in universities, in industries, and at scientific and professional meetings in the United States, Canada, Europe, the mid-East, Asia, and South Pacific. In 1960–1961 he served as president of the Society of Engineering Psychologists, in 1963–1964 as president of the Human Factors Society, and from 1976 to 1979 as president of the International Ergonomics Association. He is the recipient of a number of honors, among them an award from the International Ergonomics Association "in recognition of outstanding contributions to ergonomics internationally" and the President's Distinguished Service Award from the Human Factors Society "for a prestigious career involving dedicated service and leadership to the human factors profession." *Dr. Chapanis, a true giant in the discipline of human factors, passed away on October 4, 2002. His insights, wisdom, and presence will be missed.*

Kenneth Dandurand, RPh, MS, is cofounder and CEO of Clinical Pharmacy Associates, Inc., and cofounder and president of MedNovations, where he leads efforts to improve the quality of medication use. He received his BS in pharmacy from Northeastern University, Boston, and completed graduate training in hospital pharmacy and business management from Oregon State University and an American Society of Health-System Pharmacists-approved residency at Good Samaritan Hospital in Portland, Oregon. His clinical pharmacy experience includes community, hospital, and managed care settings. Mr. Dandurand has initiated innovative professional programs including extensive clinical pharmacy and drug information service and has spearheaded the development of models for standardized pharmacoeconomic analyses and quality improvement tools to improve the medication use process. He has served on national pharmacy and therapeutics committees for Rx Management and Pharmacy Direct Network. Mr. Dandurand has published his clinical research, currently holds an adjunct faculty appointment at Howard University College of Pharmacy, Nursing and Allied Health Science, and was a clinical faculty member of the Joint Commission on Accreditation of Healthcare Organizations (JCAHO).

Yoel Donchin, MD, is professor of anesthesia and critical care medicine at the Hadassah Hebrew University Medical School, Jerusalem, Israel. He received his MD from there in 1970 with a specialty in anesthesia. Since 1985, he has been deeply involved in the two common causes of death and disability—trauma, and human errors in the hospital. Dr. Donchin is the founder and head of the first trauma unit in Israel. During his 1990 sabbatical, he enrolled in the Department of Human Factors Engineering at the Technion, the Israeli institute of technology. With this group, he studied the nature and causes of human error in hospitals' intensive care units as well as gaps in communication among the various medical teams. Dr. Donchin served as the medical director of the Israeli Emergency Medical Service (EMS), analyzed the interior design of ambulances, and introduced safety programs for paramedics. He conducted research with the Department of Forensic Identification of the Israeli police, primarily in latent fingerprints identification and the use of postmortem computed tomographic (CT) scan for murder investigation. In 2000 he organized a course in patient safety for the medical profession in Israel. At that course, Dr. Donchin planted the seeds for the Israel National Patient Safety Foundation. He frequently publishes articles on hospital safety and accident investigation in the Israeli daily newspaper Haaretz, the Hebrew equivalent to the *New York Times*. His book, *Saving Life With First Aid,* published by the Israel Ministry of Defense Publishing House in 1997, is the official textbook on the topic in the Israeli Defense Force and the Israeli EMS or MDA. His books *A Guide to Forensic Science For Lawyers* and *Guidelines For Resuscitation* were published in Hebrew in 2001 by CARTA. Dr. Donchin currently is director of the new Patient Safety Unit at Hadassah—the first in Israel.

Maher El-Masri, PhD, is an assistant professor at the University of Windsor, Ontario, Canada. He was at the University of Maryland, School of Nursing,

Baltimore, Maryland, as a research associate with Dr. Korniewicz when he completed several research projects related to nosocomial infections and adverse effects of medical devices. His doctoral dissertation ws "Predictors of nosocomial bloodstream infections among critically ill trauma patients," which was fully funded by two grants from the American Association of Critical Care Nurses and the Pi chapter of Sigma Theta Tau. His clinical background includes several years of critical care nursing and clinical instruction in medical-surgical nursing.

Jennifer A. Ibbotson, BSc, MHK, completed a Master's in the School of Human Kinetics at the University of British Columbia after her BSc in Kinesiology at Simon Fraser University During her time at Simon Fraser University, she spent three semesters of co-operative education work placements, then part-time and full-time employment working with Dr. Christine MacKenzie in the Human Motor Systems Laboratory. She worked on the "Remote Manipulation In Endoscopic Surgery" and "Intelligent Tools for Health Care" projects, which looked at issues surrounding laparoscopic surgery. Ms. Ibbotson currently works as a research scientist in the Ergonomics and Safety Laboratory at the University of Washington.

Denise Korniewicz, DNSc, RN, FAAN, is professor, Associate Dean for Research and Doctoral Programs, and Director of the Center of Nursing Research at the University of Miami School of Nursing, Coral Gables, Florida. She has completed research on a variety of medical devices related to infection control. Her primary research has been in the area of adverse events associated with health care worker safety and patient events. She has completed both laboratory and clinical research on gloves used to protect patients and health care workers against blood-borne pathogens. Dr. Korniewicz provides consultation about infection control practices to health care facilities, attorneys, professional health care organizations, and the media. Prior to employment at the University of Maryland, she was Associate Dean for Academic Development at Georgetown University, School of Nursing, Washington, DC, Director of Adult Health at the Johns Hopkins University, School of Nursing in Baltimore, Maryland, Director of the Adult Nurse Practitioner Program at East Carolina University, Greenville, North Carolina, and served 4 years in the U.S. Army Nurse Corps. She has written numerous research articles related to clinical practice issues on patient and health care worker safety. She is a Fellow in the American Academy of Nursing. She has a BS, MS, and DNSc in nursing and completed postdoctoral education at the Johns Hopkins University, Baltimore, Maryland. She continues to do research and various speaking engagements at local, national and international conferences.

Jeanne Linden, MD, MPH, is Director, Blood and Tissue Resources for the New York State Department of Health. In this position, she oversees the activities of the blood banks and tissue banks that operate in New York. She has written several articles addressing error in transfusion medicine. She also has interest in, and has published in, the field of transfusion-transmitted diseases. Board certified in clinical pathology and transfusion medicine, she is a fellow of the College of American Pathologists. She holds a BS in chemistry from Union College, and both a Master's of Public Health and an MD from the University of Connecticut School of Medicine. She currently serves on the U.S Department of Health and Human Services Advisory Committee on Blood Safety and Availability and previously served on the U.S. Food and Drug Administration Blood Products Advisory Committee.

Alan J. Lomax, MB, ChB, FRCS (Edin), FRCS (Eng), FRCSC, practiced as a general surgeon with an interest in laparoscopic surgery in British Columbia, Canada. Dr. Lomax recently retired from active surgery and is an adjunct professor in the School of Kinesiology at Simon Fraser University. His research interests include human factors in laparoscopic surgery and technology and human error in endoscopic surgery. Visual perception and visualisation technology in endoscopic surgery, in particular 3-D technology, are other areas of interest. Dr. Lomax was also a clinical instructor on the faculty of the University of British Columbia in the Division of General Surgery and has an interest in training methods and training systems for minimally invasive surgery.

Christine L. MacKenzie, BSc, MSc, PhD, a professor of kinesiology at Simon Fraser University, in Burnaby, Canada, teaches courses in Human Factors, Human Motor Systems, and Human–Computer Interaction. She researches human motor control, goal-directed movements of the hands in skilled pianists, neurological patients, users in human–computer interaction, and surgeons performing surgical procedures. She also studies human performance in augmented environments for 3-D interaction in design, surgical trainng, and collaborative activities. She published *The Grasping Hand* in 1994. Her endoscopic surgery research has been funded since 1995 by the British Columbia Health Research Foundation for "Remote Manipulation In Endoscopic Surgery" and by Canada's Network of Centres of Excellence on Robotics and Intelligent Systems' "Intelligent Tools for Health Care Project."

Colin F. Mackenzie, MD, received his medical degree from the University of Aberdeen, Scotland in 1968. He completed a residency in anesthesiology at the University of London, England, and came to the Shock Trauma Center in Baltimore in 1975. He became board certified by the American Board of Anesthesiology and was elected Fellow of the American College of Critical Care Medicine in 1990. He is a tenured professor with a joint appointment in the Departments of Anesthesiology and Physiology at the University of Maryland School of Medicine. He was formerly Chief of Trauma Anesthesiology at the Shock Trauma Center. He is Director of the Charles Mc. Mathias, Jr. National Study Center for Trauma and EMS. Dr. Mackenzie has edited three books, written more than

25 book chapters, and published over 80 peer-reviewed scientific papers. His areas of research interest include telecommunications for medicine, trauma patient resuscitation and transfusion, hemoglobin-based O_2 carrying solutions, and human factors in emergencies. He is currently funded by several federal agencies including Agency for Healthcare Research and Quality (AHRQ), National Science Foundation (NSF), National Library of Medicine (NLM), and the U.S. Army.

Ulrich Matern, MD, is a surgeon at the Department of General Surgery, University Hospital of Freiburg, Germany. He is chief of the Study Group on Surgical Technologies. This interdisciplinary group aims to improve the technical field of surgery and to build a vision of the operating room of the future. New instruments and devices are developed by the group in cooperation with industry. The current working place and the new technologies are tested and measured by different methods such as by electromyogram and video observation.

Denise Park, PhD, is Professor of Psychology and Research Scientist at the Beckman Institute at the University of Illinois. Dr. Park has an extensive research program examining the effect of age-related changes in cognition in the ability of older adults to process medical information and perform health-related activities. She has been continuously funded by the National Institute on Aging (NIA) since 1981 and directs an NIA-sponsored Roybal Center on health, cognition, and aging. She is past president of Division 20 (Adult Development and Aging) of the American Psychological Association (APA), past chair of the APA's Board of Scientific Affairs, chaired an NIH study section, and served as associate editor for the *Journal of Gerontology: Psychological Sciences* and for the *American Psychologist.* In addition to her interests in health, cognition, and aging, Dr. Park is also interested in brain–behavior relationships and functional neuroimaging, as well as the interaction of culture, aging, and cognition. She has edited several books and published numerous articles on these topics.

Penelope Sanderson, PhD, is Professor of Cognitive Engineering and Human Factors at the Australian Research Council's Key Centre for Human Factors and Applied Cognitive Psychology at The University of Queensland in Brisbane, Australia. Professor Sanderson received her BA(Honors) in 1979 from University of Western Australia and her MA in 1982 and PhD in 1985 from the University of Toronto. She was on the faculty at the University of Illinois at Urbana-Champaign for 11 years before returning to Australia in 1997 to take up the inaugural directorship of the Swinburne Computer Human Interaction Laboratory at Swinburne University in Melbourne. Professor Sanderson's research in medical human factors covers the design of visual and auditory displays for anesthesia and intensive care environments. She has served on the editorial board of *Human Factors* and currently is on the editorial board of *Cognition, Technology, and Work.* From 1997 to 1998 she served as chair of the Medical

Systems and Rehabilitation Technical Group of the Human Factors and Ergonomics Society. In 1996 Professor Sanderson qualified as a licensed emergency medical technician in the state of Illinois.

F. Jacob Seagull, PhD, is an assistant professor in the University of Maryland Department of Anesthesiology. He is involved in research regarding the effects of various technologies on human performance within the domain of medical care provision, such as telemedicine and advanced displays for anesthesiology. He is also Patient Safety Scientist in the University of Maryland Medical System, working with the Patient Safety Team, which is responsible for improving patient safety throughout the university's medical system. He received his PhD in psychology from the University of Illinois at Urbana-Champaign, focusing his research on the problems of alarms in anesthesia. He received his BA with high honors in psychology from the University of Michigan and his MS in engineering psychology and behavioral sciences from the Technion—Israel's institute of technology. He has carried out research in attentional aspects of helmet-mounted displays, human–computer interaction, and alarms systems in medical devices. His research interests include patient safety, human perception and performance, and cognitive engineering.

Ian Skurnik, PhD, is an assistant professor of marketing at the University of Toronto. He completed his PhD at Princeton University in social psychology and a postdoctoral fellowship sponsored by the National Institute on Aging at the University of Michigan. He has interests in the illusion of truth and how it affects medical errors, as well as memory for advertisements.

Matthew B. Weinger, MD, is Professor of Anesthesiology at the University of California San Diego and a staff physician in the VA San Diego Healthcare System. He is the director of the San Diego Center for Patient Safety, and runs its Center for Healthcare Simulation. Dr. Weinger received a BS degree in electrical engineering and an MS in biological sciences from Stanford University in 1978. He received an M.D. degree in 1982 at the University of California San Diego and became a board-certified anesthesiologist after receiving clinical training at the University of California San Francisco. Currently, Dr. Weinger provides anesthesia to patients, teaches undergraduate and graduate students and physicians, and conducts human factors research in anesthesia and critical care medicine. Over the last 15 years, Dr. Weinger has published more than 85 articles and chapters, given numerous invited presentations, and been awarded several million dollars in research grants. He teaches classes on decision making and patient safety. He is the co-chairman of the Association for the Advancement of Medical Instrumentation (AAMI) Human Factors Engineering Committee that is developing American national standards for the design of medical device user interfaces. He is also a member of the board of directors of the Anesthesia Patient Safety Foundation and a past president of the Society for Technology in Anesthesia.

Yan Xiao, PhD, directs the Human Factors & Technology Research at the University of Maryland School of Medicine and is the principal investigator of six major projects, totaling $2.8 million, funded by federal agencies and Fortune 100 companies. Among his contributions are innovative designs of mobile tele-medicine systems, theories of collaborative work, and designs of effective audi-tory alarms in health care. He is a member of peer-review panels for grant appli-cations for the National Science Foundation and National Aeronautical and Space Administration. His work on telemedicine has also been reported in trade magazines and television documentaries. Currently Dr. Xiao is associate profes-sor (tenured) of anesthesiology and information systems and a special member of the faculty in the School of Business, University of Maryland, College Park. Yan Xiao has a PhD in Human Factors from University of Toronto (1994). He also has a MASc in Systems Engineering (1985, Beijing Institute of Technol-ogy) and BASc in Mechanical Engineering (1982, Lanzhou Railway Univer-sity). His current work has been in the following three areas: efficiency and patient safety, establishing principles of telecommunication, and coordination. Major sponsors of his research include the National Patient Safety Foundation, National Institutes of Health, National Science Foundation, Army Research Institute, and Nortel Networks.

1 Understanding Human Error

Marilyn Sue Bogner
Institute for the Study of Human Error, LLC

> It is one thing to show a man that he is in an error,
> and another to put him in possession of truth.
>
> —John Locke (1632–1704)
> *An Essay Concerning Human Understanding*

In all aspects of life, human error has been the attributed cause of faulty products and accidents with consequences ranging from inconvenience, through loss of property and resources, to death. The media informs the public of disasters caused by human error. Among those disasters are the collapse of crowded walkways in the Kansas City Hyatt Regency Hotel (114 people killed and 200 injured) due to a deviation in the structural design and unanticipated use (Petroski, 1992); the sinking of the ferry *Herald of Free Enterprise* (188 crew and passengers lost) because the bow doors through which cars entered were not closed, allowing the ocean to enter the hold (Buck, 1989), and the emissions from the Chernobyl nuclear power plant failure that were carried by the winds to affect distant communities. People express interest and concern about those incidents as well as other construction, transportation, and industrial disasters reported as caused by human error. There is no hue and cry, however, for something to be done about them. After all, those disasters happened to other people in other places—they didn't affect us. Then came the bombshell of a report on human error that affects everyone.

The population of the United States was, shocked, stunned, and outraged by the Institute of Medicine's (IOM) report, *To Err Is Human,* which cited human error in medicine as the cause of death for tens of thousands of individuals who sought the curative powers of hospitalized care (Kohn, Corrigan, & Donaldson, 1999). Close on the heels of that report was one from the United Kingdom (U.K.) indicating that in National Health Service hospitals medical errors harm (inflict injury as well as death to) 10% of admissions, or a rate in excess of 850,000 annually (Department of Health, 2000). Although the U.K. report received a pittance of the media coverage of the IOM report, it gave credence to the number of deaths attributed to human error by the IOM.

Not only did the U.K. report confirm that medical error is a problem, by including injuries as well as deaths in the reported number, it also expanded the magnitude of the problem. The numbers cited in the IOM report were of deaths; including error-related injuries would increase the numbers considerably. Although it has not been assessed, there is no reason to doubt that harm related to errors also occurs in outpatient care, which increases the magnitude of the problem even more. The problem would be even greater if, in addition to serious injuries and death, the number of patients who require additional treatment because of adverse outcomes from error were included. Thus, medical error or, more broadly stated to include all forms of care, health care error is a problem—a problem with profound financial and social implications for the nation at large as well as ramifications for the people directly involved.

To address the problem of medical error, the IOM report recommended a mandatory adverse event reporting program that requires health care providers, particularly physicians, to report their errors for the purpose of accountability. That recommendation reflects the assumption about the nature of error expressed in the title of the IOM report, an attitude that is pervasive throughout society, that humans, including health care providers, are innately error-prone. Such an attitude is very powerful because it determines the focus of efforts to reduce the likelihood of error. If the focus is accurate, then efforts to address error are effective; however, if the focus is inappropriate, then efforts to address error are misdirected and the problem persists. To address adverse outcomes through appropriately directed efforts, it is necessary to understand human error. The first step in understanding human error is to define it.

DEFINING ERROR

Typically an error is described in terms of what happened, the adverse outcome such as amputating a healthy leg, making an inaccurate diagnosis, omitting a dose of medication, or more generally, deviating from the standard of care. The commonality in those examples is that each involves an act, an action by a care provider that affects the patient. This can be an act of commission, an overt activity, or an act of omission, the absence of an activity. In addition, an error may be rule-based, skill-based, or knowledge-based (Rasmussen, 1990a). Errors can be slips, lapses, mistakes, and violations; they can occur at the sharp end, immediate to, and at the blunt end, distant from, the point of care as well as be latent (Reason, 1990). Although the variety of descriptions indicates that errors have differing characteristics, they all describe acts, behaviors.

ERROR AS BEHAVIOR

Considering error as behavior is important to understanding human error. It bridges the real world of health care errors with the nearly two centuries of insights from the academic discipline that studies human behavior, psychology, as well as the many centuries of thought on the human condition by psychology's parent, philosophy. Error as behavior also is the bridge to insights expressed in plays, novels, biographies, and other writings by astute observers of human endeavors—insights that can aide in understanding human error as discussed in the last chapter of this book.

Theory and research findings describe human behavior as the interaction of the person and the environment. The extent to which a person influences the environment and is influenced by it varies by school of thought; nonetheless, the insight provided for understanding error is that behavior is a function not of a person in isolation, but of the person interacting with the environment (Lewin, 1936/1966). This expands the understanding of error from the simple concept of people committing errors driven by their innate error-proneness, to the complexity of people interacting with their vast and varied environments. To appreciate the importance of this expansion, let us consider what is involved in the delivery of health care.

Health Care Delivery

Human error in health care typically is considered as just that, an error committed by a person, an error-prone human. This concept is reflected in programs that require care providers to report their errors. An error reported as an adverse outcome is a solitary data point. An outcome, however, is not a disembodied datum; an outcome doesn't happen spontaneously. Rather, an outcome is the result of a treatment administered by the provider such as a medical procedure, a diagnosis, a test, counseling—an error involves a means of providing care. An error happens to a person, the care recipient—an error involves a patient. Thus, what began as a seemingly simple concept of error in terms of only an adverse outcome has become a complex concept involving the provider, the means of providing care, and the care recipient. Health care is not static; for an outcome to occur some activity must take place. That activity involves interactions among the three entities, which increases the complexity of the concept of error.

Even though a health care provider interacts with the means of providing care and with the patient, little attention is paid to possible implications for provider performance from the means of providing care and even less to implications from the care recipient. There are performance implications, however; each of these entities is a system of interacting and interdependent characteristics that affect and are affected by characteristics of the others (Bogner, 1998). The health of a care provider influences how a technologically sophisticated means of providing care is applied to a morbidly obese patient; changes in any of the entities can cause changes in the others. Such interrelated and interdependent interactions define a system; hence, the three systems involved in the delivery of health care become subsystems of the basic care providing system (Bogner, 1998).

Because the interaction of the characteristics of the members of the basic unit of health care delivery define a system, understanding provider error necessarily involves the consideration of error in terms of the members of that system: the means of providing care and the care recipient. The discussion to this point has addressed health care delivery devoid of environmental context; yet it does occur in a context.

Environmental Context

In no other human endeavor do a wider variety of people perform tasks in more diverse conditions than in health care. Health care is delivered by professionals skilled in a wide range of specialties, athletic trainers, medics, and lay persons ranging from the elderly to children; health care is delivered in hospitals, on sports fields, in space modules, on battlefields, and in the work place. Errors can and do occur in all of these contexts. Although the IOM report (Kohn, Corrigan, & Donaldson, 1999) and that regarding the National Health Service in the U.K. (Department of Health, 2000) address error by health care professionals in hospital settings, consideration of other environmental contexts of health care— contexts in which errors and adverse outcomes occur, can provide broadly applicable insights. The complexity of the greater environment even as it applies to hospitals presents a challenge for understanding error; the magnitude of the problem of adverse health care outcomes demands that the challenge be met. Assistance in meeting that challenge comes from industry.

LESSONS LEARNED FROM INDUSTRY

Factors have been identified that affect the performance of a person and lead to error in industries such as nuclear power and manufacturing (Moray, 1994; Rasmussen, 1982, 1994; Senders & Moray, 1991). Admittedly, health care is not the same as the activities of those industries, however, to the extent that such evidence-based factors may contribute to error in general, considering them with respect to health care could lead to insights vital to understanding human error whether it occurs in industry or health care.

Factors identified as contributing to errors in specific industries when extrapolated from those industries can be considered as factors in the general environmental context of a task that contribute to error. Those factors are clustered into five categories representing aspects of the context of care (Bogner, 2000).

Context of Care

The factors in each of the categories of the aspects of the context of care are interrelated; they affect and are affected by the other factors in the specific category. By being interrelated, the factors in each category define the category as a system. These categories of factors are the five systems of the context of care: ambient conditions, physical environment, social environment, organizational factors, and the overarching legal-regulatory-reimbursement-national culture factors represented as the concentric circles in Fig. 1.1. The five systems are interrelated and interdependent and as such define the context of care as a system.

The three systems of the basic care-providing system, the provider, means of providing care, and the care recipient, are embedded in the system of the context of care. Those eight systems of factors are interrelated and interdependent and define the overall context of error as a system. In keeping with the food analogies of error as Swiss cheese (Reason, 1990), and an onion (Moray, 1994), this systems approach to error (Bogner, 2000) is analogous to an artichoke. The leaves of the artichoke are the concentric circles in Fig. 1.1 representing the five contextual systems, with the system of overarching factors being the external leaves and each system of characteristics, the organizational factors, social environment, physical environment, and ambient conditions as concentric rings of leaves surrounding the heart of the artichoke, the basic care providing system.

The concept of the context of error as a system of subsystems is important in considering the impact of factors on provider performance, hence error. Changes in any of the systems of the context of error produce a reverse ripple. Rather than rippling out from the point of impact, as when the surface of a pond

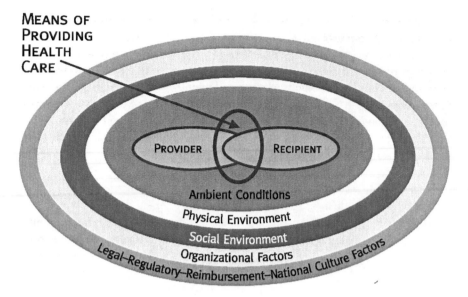

MEANS OF
PROVIDING
HEALTH
CARE

PROVIDER   RECIPIENT

Ambient Conditions
Physical Environment
Social Environment
Organizational Factors
Legal–Regulatory–Reimbursement–National Culture Factors

FIG. 1.1.   The systems approach artichoke model of error.

is disturbed by a stone, the impact of a change in any system ripples inward. That is, systems within the circumference of the system with the change are influenced by the change (see Fig. 1.1). For example, changes in the physical environment affect the social environment, ambient conditions, and ultimately the members of the basic care providing system, the care provider, means of providing care, and the patient with little if any impact on the organization and none on the overarching societal level factors.

The greatest impact occurs from a change in the overarching system of legal-regulatory-reimbursement-national culture factors. A change in reimbursement policies that reduces the amount of reimbursement for certain procedures alters the funds available to the organization which necessitates reductions such as the number and educational level of the staff; this affects communication among the staff and with patients' families, building maintenance, purchasing of equipment, and patients who present at more advanced stages of illness—all of which affect the care provider.

Because of the reverse ripple, the origin of a factor that induces error may be other than where the factor impacts the provider, so efforts to change those factors may be applied inappropriately and doomed to failure. For example, a resident's excessive workload although emanating from the organization, the hospital, may be the result of funding limited by reimbursement policies. Directing the hospital to reduce the workload could be ineffective or even counterproductive; efforts would be directed more appropriately to those governing reimbursement policies.

In terms of the artichoke model, exerting strong pressure on a leaf in one of the circles of leaves representing systems results in pressure which changes the condition of circles of leaves, the systems, between the ring where the leaf is pressured and the heart of the artichoke. The basic system of care, by being central to the context of care, is affected by a change in any system; the heart of the artichoke is affected by what happens to any of the leaves.

WHY BLAME THE PROVIDER?

The meaning of a sentence is questioned when it is taken out of context, contexts are constructed with soft light and music to evoke certain behaviors, and efforts are made to construct the social context of a society from its archaeological artifacts. Yet, the context in which a health care error occurs typically is not considered as playing a role in the error; the care provider is blamed for the error. It is acknowledged that care providers commit errors; however, blame provides no insights as to why the error occurred so that it may be prevented, no aid in understanding human error. Thus the question, why blame the provider?

In addressing an event such as an error, people tend to seek a reasonable explanation for it, and once such an explanation or cause is identified, the search for a reason for the event goes no further. The exercise of this stop rule (Rasmussen, 1990b) that terminates the search for a reasonable explanation for an adverse outcome in health care at the care provider can be the reflection of the prevailing attitude that people are inherently error prone. This has a profound affect on the interpretation of adverse events, hence the understanding of human error.

Interpretation of Adverse Events

The influence of attitudes on the interpretation of behavior is pervasive. The actions of a person are interpreted to be in harmony with the interpreter's attitude toward those actions or toward the person (Heider, 1958); that is, if Person A has the attitude that Person B is honest, then B's words and deeds will be interpreted by A as honest. Similarly, if a person has the attitude that people are error-prone, when considering an adverse event, the reasonable explanation for that event is an error by a person. The subtle impact of this attitude on interpreting adverse events is illustrated by several examples.

The power of the stop rule is apparent in the identification of errors using infusion pumps (computer chip driven devices that are programmed to regulate the flow of fluid into the body) and parenteral delivery devices (the programmed delivery of nutritional fluids into a person via an infusion-pump-like device). The identified errors involved programming pumps, accidental tubing discon- nections, and confusion between central and peripheral lines (Leape et al., 1995). The responsibility for those problems is implicitly yet clearly stated; the problems were caused by the people using the device. The attitude that humans are error-prone is so subtle and pervasive that there may seem to be no other explanation; however, from the discussion of the basic care providing system, we know there can be other explanations.

Not evoking the stop rule based on the attitude that humans are inherently error-prone allows the consideration of factors in the context of error as possible explanations. This leads to explaining the problems in terms of the design of the pumps that make them difficult to program (Brown, Bogner, Parmentier, & Tay- lor, 1997), have connections that are loose so they spontaneously disconnect, and have identical appearing, difficult-to-differentiate central and peripheral lines (Bogner, 2002). Exercising the stop rule at the care provider for problems with infusion pumps typically results in subjecting care providers to training or other efforts to improve their performance. Because those efforts do not address the source of the problem, the design of the pump, the problem persists and adverse events are repeated.

Another example is reporting of adverse drug events as the result of physician ordering, nurse administration, transcription, and pharmacy dispensing (Leape et al., 1995). If the stop rule that people are the source of errors were not evoked and the means of providing care considered, the interpretation would be *drug* ordering, *drug* administration, transcription, and *drug* dispensing (Bogner, 2002). This latter expression of the findings focuses attention to the drug involved, such as Celebrex® being substituted for Celexa®. Identifying the care providers as the cause of the problem eclipses the error-provoking factor of look-alike drug names—a factor that will continue to cause confusion unless the focus is removed from care providers and placed on the actual contributing factor so efforts to address the error can be effective.

When considering the adverse outcome of infection at the site of a surgical procedure, the typical reasonable explanation is error by one of the surgical team members. To reduce that error, surgical team members are required to attend training. If the stop rule were not evoked at the point of persons and the search for the explanation of the infection continued, the analysis might have found that the cold ambient temperature in the operating room encourages infection (Buggy, 2000; Kurz, Sessler, & Lenhardt, 1996). The premature identification of the source of the problem as people and subsequent remedial action directed to them allows the infection-inducing conditions to persist and the cycle of patients acquiring infections, care providers being blamed for the infections, and training to change performance is perpetuated.

As with the infusion pumps, drug error, and surgical infection examples, the attitude that people cause errors leads to evoking the stop rule to identify care providers as sources of the errors, whereas the factors that actually contribute to the errors reside beyond the care provider in the context of error. The systems approach model is a useful tool for understanding error because it promotes examination of each system for error-inducing factors; hence it forces the suspension of the stop rule.

The insight that error behavior reflects the person acting upon and reacting to, thus being influenced by, factors in the environment points to the inappropriateness of the attitude that to err is human. That attitude could give the impression that humans alone are prone to error and prevent possible insights for understanding human error.

LESSONS OF THE DRUG VIAL, THE FLY, THE DOG, AND THE HARD-WIRED CAPABILITIES OF THE HUMAN

If the person is acted upon by the environment and commits an error, then although the erroneous act actually is made by the person, the influence of the error-provoking factors, rather than the error-prone nature of the person alone, contributed to the act. This is not to deny that the person committing the error is accountable for it, but to determine why the error occurred. The error provoking influence of factors in the environment is illustrated by three examples, two of which indicate that error is not a uniquely human accomplishment.

Two vials of drugs were placed side by side in an area where doses of medications were being prepared. The vials were the same size with the same color tops and the same size labels with similar constellations of letters indicating the drug names—labels that looked alike *except* that the name of one drug ended in "en" and the name of the other ended in "on." It was night, and the light was dim in the area; the care provider, who had not had his vision checked since his last driver's license renewal 4 years earlier, drew up the drug with the name ending in "on" instead of the one with "en" and injected the patient. The patient experienced distress that was not life threatening and recovered fully. Thus, the provider committed an error. He did, but at the instigation of error-inducing factors.

Insects and animals typically are not considered as error-prone beings; however, that is not the case. Many varieties of flies are attracted to the odor of carrion; they lay their eggs on it so the larvae have food when they hatch. Those flies also are attracted to the carrion odor emitted by certain plants and lay their eggs on the plant leaves, presuming that to be source of nutrition for the larvae based on the emitted odor. The odor-emitting plant does not provide food for the larvae; as a result of the fly's error, the larvae die (Mach, 1905/1976). Non-human error is not unique to the lowly fly.

It is not unusual for people, when standing engaged in conversation at a social gathering such as a cookout, to find themselves standing ever closer to their neighbor as they deftly although erroneously are herded into a small cluster by the family's diligent Australian sheepdog. Sheepdogs have been observed doing what has been considered as nearly impossible—herding cats! People are not sheep; indeed they are two-legged, not four-legged, beings. Cats are not sheep by physiognomy and certainly not by overt disposition even though they have four legs. Apparently, these differentiations are not sufficient to discourage a sheepdog, ever vigilant for opportunities to exercise his skills, from committing errors in selecting subjects for herding. People and cats, as well as sheep, are mobile beings and as such are targets for the sheepdog's efforts.

The inappropriate interaction with the environment by the health care provider may be considered as a manifestation of the human's propensity to err. This might be addressed by training to observe drug names or the implementation of a policy requiring that the name of every drug be read three times before administering it. What of the fly? Should she be trained to better differentiate real carrion from a plant, or might the aspect of the environment, the odor from the plant, be considered an environmental factor that elicits error behavior? What of the dog? Should he be trained to differentiate people and cats from sheep, or is the presence of mobile beings in his environment a factor that triggers his behavior, as inappropriate as it may be for the people and certainly for the cats involved?

If the presence of environmental factors is a reasonable explanation for the error behavior of the fly and the dog, then although humans are purported to be higher order beings than flies and dogs, the environmental factor of the look-alike vials and drug names might be a reasonable explanation for the error by the care provider. The characteristics of the environmental factors in each of the three examples are common, suggesting a compelling error-inducing factor. The factor is similarity—of vial, label, and drug name, of odor, of mobile beings. Indeed, the characteristic of similarity has been documented as force in human perception (Kohler, 1929)—a force that can cause confused identification.

The lessons of the drug vial, the fly and the dog suggest that certain potential error-inducing propensities are inherent in organisms and as such are not amenable to change through training, policy, or chastisement; in technological terms, there are propensities and capabilities that are hard-wired in an individual and not amenable to programming, regardless of the number and variety of attempts to do so. Among the number of capabilities directly affecting the study of medical error and patient safety that are hard-wired in the human in addition to similarity, is the capability for actively retaining and considering information (Eysenck, 1984).

Although it is well known and documented that the human capability for dealing with information is limited, industry develops technologically sophisticated medical devices—ever pushing the envelope of technology—many of which provide information far in excess of what a person can assimilate at a given time. Some critical care units have multiple devices that provide information in excess of the human's hard-wired capability to comprehend. An implicit assumption exists that health care providers can adjust to any set of circumstances, including the demands of a medical device. Indeed, care providers may be able to chain the bits of information to accommodate more, but that capability also is limited by the way the human is hard-wired.

A manual accompanies a cognitively demanding device and in-service training may be provided. It is assumed, although not tested, that the intended user will be able to use the device effectively from reading the manual and attending the training, even though the demands of the device surpass human capability. If an adverse outcome occurs because information was not assimilated, it typically is considered the fault of the care provider. Thus, working conditions that ignore hard-wired human capabilities can and will provoke error. If error is to be prevented, the complexity of the task must be matched with the complexity and the hard-wired capabilities of the person to perform the task (Weick, 1987).

GATHERING THE PIECES OF THE PUZZLE OF HUMAN ERROR

Health care providers indeed do commit errors, but that is not proof of innate error-producing proclivities of humans. In terms of the quote from Locke at the beginning of this chapter, it shows that people are in an error. To possess the truth of error, to understand human error, it is necessary to determine why the error occurred. The perspective of the health care provider is central to that determination. Considering error solely in terms of the person addresses only some of the contributing factors, only pieces of the puzzle that is human error. Without all of the pieces, the picture of the error is incomplete and misleading. Understanding error as behavior that involves the person interacting with the environment can provide missing pieces of the puzzle; however, to do so, the picture of the puzzle should be through the window of the perspective of the involved care provider. The picture of factors in the context of error that affected the behavior of the provider at the time of the adverse event allows the identification of factors that contributed to, induced, and provoked error. That picture contributes to understanding human error.

REFERENCES

Bogner, M. S. (1998, October). Error: It's what, not who. *TraumaCare, 8*(2), 82–84.

Bogner, M. S. (2000). A systems approach to medical error. In C. Vincent & B. De Mol (Eds.), *Safety in medicine* (pp. 83–101). Amsterdam: Pergamon.

Bogner, M. S. (2002, Spring). Stretching the search for the "why" of error: The systems approach. *Journal of Clinical Engineering, 27*(2), 110–115.

Brown, S. L., Bogner, M. S., Parmentier, C. M., & Taylor, J. B. (1997). Human error and patient-controlled analgesia pumps. *Journal of Intravenous Nursing, 20,* 311–317.

Buck, L. (1989, September). Human error at sea. *Human Factors Society Bulletin, 32*(9), 12.

Buggy, D. (2000, July 29). Can anaesthetic management influence surgical-wound healing? *The Lancet, 356,* 355–356.

Department of Health. (2000). *An organization with a memory: Report of an expert group on learning from adverse events in the National Health Service.* Norwich, UK: The Stationery Office.

Eysenck, M. W. (1984. *A handbook of cognitive psychology.* Hillsdale, NJ: Lawrence Erlbaum Associates.

Heider, F. (1958). *The psychology of interpersonal relations.* New York: John Wiley & Sons, Inc.

Kohn, L. T., Corrigan, J. M., & Donaldson, M. S. (Eds.). (1999). *To err is human: Building a safer health care system.* Washington, DC: National Academy Press.

Kohler, W. (1929). *Gestalt psychology.* New York: Boni & Liveright.

Kurz, A. K, Sessler, D. I., & Lenhardt, R. (1996). Perioperative normothermia to reduce the incidence of surgical-wound infection and shorten hospitalization. *New England Journal of Medicine, 334,* 1209–1215.

Leape, L. L., Bates, D. W., Cullen, D. J., Cooper, J., Demonaco, H. J., Gallivan, T., Hallisay, R., Ives, J., Laird, N., Laffel, G., Nemeskal, N., Petersen, L. A., Porter, J., Servi, D., Shea, B. F., Small, S., Sweitzer, B., Thompson, B. T., & Vander Vliet, M. (1995). Systems analysis of adverse drug events. *Journal of the American Medical Association, 274,* 35–43.

Lewin, K. (1966). *Principles of topological psychology.* New York: McGraw-Hill.

Moray, N. (1994). Error reduction as a systems problem. In M. S. Bogner (Ed.), *Human error in medicine* (pp. 67–91). Mahwah, NJ: Lawrence Erlbaum Associates.

Mach, E. (1976). *Knowledge and error.* Dordrecht-Holland: D. Reidel.

Petroski, H. (1992). *To engineer is human.* New York: Vintage Books.

Rasmussen, J. (1982). Human errors: A taxonomy for describing human malfunction in industrial installations. *Journal of Occupational Accidents, 4,* 311–333.

Rasmussen, J. (1990a). The role of error in organizing behavior. *Ergonomics, 33,* 1185–1190.

Rasmussen, J. (1990b). Human error and the problem of causality in analysis of accidents. *Philosophical Transactions of the Royal Society of London, B 327,* 449–462.

Rasmussen, J. (1994). Afterword. In M. S. Bogner (Ed.) *Human error in medicine* (pp. 385–394). Mahwah, NJ: Lawrence Erlbaum Associates.

Reason, J. T. (1990). *Human error.* New York: Cambridge University Press.

Senders, J. W., & Moray, N. P. (1991). *Human error: Cause, prediction, and reduction.* Mahwah, NJ: Lawrence Erlbaum Associates.

Soukhanov, A. H., & Ellis, K. (Eds.) (1994). *Webster's II New Riverside University Dictionary.* New York: The Riverside Publishing Company

Weick, K. E. (1987). Organizational culture as a source of high reliability. *California Management Review, 29,* 112–127.

2

The Trouble With Blood Is It All Looks the Same: Transfusion Errors

Jeanne V. Linden
New York State Department of Health

BLOOD BANK TECHNOLOGIST, LAURA PETERSON SURGICAL INTENSIVE CARE NURSE, SHIRLEY BROWN SURGICAL RESIDENT, BRUCE JONES, M.D.

Sam Cohen loved his job as a paramedic. It offered the opportunity to truly help people in time of need and posed diverse challenges every day. It also posed a contrast to his stable personal life. He had dated his wife, Donna, when they were in high school, and they had married a few years later. Their sons, Brian, age 6, and Jeremy, age 4, were the joy of their life. Raising children in an urban setting was a challenge, but Sam always made it a point to take them to the park on his one weekend day off.

One beautiful summer morning, Sam was jogging along the edge of the park, which was his usual routine. He heard a large truck approach from behind him. It suddenly jumped the curb and Sam was unable to get out of the way in time. He looked up at the truck's grill and then everything went black.

In the emergency department of Liberty Hospital, emergency medicine physician George Johnson had just come on duty. With the good weather, he hoped it would be a quiet day. He was going to get a cup of coffee when paramedics wheeled in a man who looked to be about 30, dressed in jogging shorts and a T-shirt, covered with blood. After examination, George determined that the patient had open fractures of one arm and both legs and also had free blood in his abdomen. Because the man had no identification, he was assigned an identifier, WM, the next in the sequence of initials used. A wristband with this identifier, together with a medical record number, 687115, was placed on his undamaged arm.

Patient WM, 687115 was sent to the operating room where opening his abdomen revealed several lacerations of the liver, laceration of his colon, and free blood in the abdomen. The liver lacerations were repaired, the damaged intestine was removed, and the remaining intestine was sewn back together. During the surgery, blood lost was suctioned and cleaned through a blood recovery device and re-infused. Because the man had been under anesthesia for several hours, the plan was to take him back to the operating room the following day to set the fractures surgically. Following the abdominal surgery, he was taken to the surgical intensive care unit. Laboratory testing showed that his blood count was very low—21% (about half of normal for a man), which was consistent with extensive blood loss. He would need blood transfusions. It is customary for physicians to order that blood be crossmatched—a procedure to determine the compatibility of the patient's blood with the blood intended to be transfused—prior to anticipated need and held so it will be available when needed. Two units of banked blood were ordered to be tested and crossmatched for patient WM, 687115. A sample of his blood was sent to the blood bank to implement that order.

Laura Peterson usually worked in clinical chemistry, but was covering the blood bank because the person who typically worked there was home ill. Laura had been trained in blood bank procedures, but did not perform them very often. Her first task when she received the blood sample labeled WM, 687115 was to test it to determine its type. There are four blood types based on the presence or absence of two antigens, A and B; they are types O, A, B, and AB. People with blood type A or B have one antigen, type AB people have both, and type O people have neither. Thus, type A blood presents a foreign antigen that type O patients and type B patients lack and can respond to with an immune response— antibodies that attack and destroy cells containing the foreign antigen. Likewise, B is a foreign antigen for type O and type A patients.

Laura determined that the sample from WM, 687115 was type O. She also crossmatched that sample of blood with donor units. This involved mixing some of the patient's blood in a test tube with a sample of that to be transfused to see if there is a reaction—a test that mimics the type of interaction that would occur in the patient's body. After crossmatching, Laura labeled the units and set them on a shelf in the refrigerator.

Shortly after receiving the sample from WM, 687115, Laura received a sample of blood from patient WN, 687116. She typed that sample and found it to be type A. She crossmatched the blood from that patient, attached an identification tag to the units and set them on the refrigerator shelf next to those for patient WM, 687115. There was a lot of surgery scheduled that day and a flurry of demand for blood bank services. Laura was very busy with a number of blood samples for typing and crossmatching.

The request came for the two units of red blood cells for patient WM, 687115. Laura responded by starting to prepare the units for release. This preparation entails removing the units from the refrigerator and comparing the tie tag on each unit with the intended patient's identifying information. As Laura was attaching the tags, the telephone rang with an urgent request from the operating room for blood for a surgical patient who was bleeding. She prepared and released those units to the operating room. Before releasing any units, Laura was to enter the activity in the computer. The computer's software was designed not only to record what blood is released, but also to verify that the type of the blood released and the blood of the patient are compatible. Laura had received training in the use of the computer, but had not become comfortable with using it; to her, it was quite cumbersome. The manual release procedures were faster than using the computer for Laura. With a backlog of several pending requests for blood, saving time was important, so Laura did not enter the activity in the computer when she released a unit for patient WM, 687115. In her rush, Laura did not match the patient's assigned name, represented by letters and ID number, carefully with the information on the unit tag. Inadvertently, without knowing it, Laura released one of the group A units intended for patient WN, 687116 to patient WM, 687115.

Shirley Brown enjoyed working as a nurse in the surgical intensive care unit (SICU). The patients were very sick in the SICU, which provided her a good opportunity to really help them. Shirley felt sorry for the young man who had been hit by a truck, but was optimistic that he would recover fully. He had just arrived from the operating room and was still unconscious. She checked his vital signs, administered the medications that had been ordered, and drew some blood for lab tests. She knew that blood had been ordered, so she was not surprised when a unit arrived. The standard operating procedure required her to compare the patient's name and identification number at the bedside with the tag on the unit of blood in the presence of another nurse for confirmation. When the unit of blood came, all the other nurses were busy as usual. Shirley wanted to expedite the young man's recovery, so she was eager for him to receive his blood as soon as possible. She decided that she would ask Becky to double check and sign for the confirmation of the blood unit later.

Although Shirley examined the identification tag on the blood unit, the identification stated in the paperwork, and name on the patient's wristband, she did not notice that the unit was identified as WN, 687116 and the wristband stated WM, 687115. Shirley hung the unit of blood for transfusion, set the flow rate, and began to monitor the patient's vital signs as the transfusion began. A few minutes after the transfusion started, the patient's blood pressure dropped 10 points and his temperature rose from 100.8 degrees to 103.8 degrees. Shirley also noticed that the urine in the patient's Foley bag, drained through an indwelling catheter, had turned pink, indicating that blood or blood cell remnants were present in the urinary tract. Although the SICU patients tended to be extremely ill, the changes exhibited by WM, 687115 were outside the usual parameters. Shirley made a mental note to follow up on these symptoms. Before she could do that, she was called to take care of a patient who had just arrived from the operating room.

When Shirley returned to patient WM, 687115, his blood pressure was lower and his temperature higher than before she left, and he was having difficulty breathing. She searched for a resident physician and located Bruce Jones, a second-year postmedical school surgical resident who was the junior resident on duty. Although Bruce had no formal instruction in administering transfusions, he was conscientious and competent in obtaining on-the-job training as a resident. He was busy with another patient. Shirley completed administration of the unit of blood, and went about administering medications to that patient and the other patients under her care. She finally was able to get talk with Bruce. She reported to him the drop in blood pressure, the fever, pink urine, and the difficulty breathing in patient WM, 687115. Bruce briefly considered the possibility of a transfusion reaction, but decided that the symptoms Shirley reported more likely were a result of the trauma.

Bruce discussed the situation by phone with his senior resident supervisor, a fifth-year postmedical school surgical resident who also had no formal training administering transfusions, but more experience than Bruce; however all of his transfusions had gone well, which limited his experience with transfusion reactions. Because patient WM, 687115 was so anemic, Bruce and his supervisor agreed that it was important for the second unit of blood be administered, so they decided not to order a transfusion reaction work-up. The work-up would have involved sending blood and urine specimens to the lab, which would have delayed the second transfusion for the patient. They elected to proceed and monitor the patient.

A second unit of blood arrived about 20 minutes later. All the other nurses were busy and unavailable to confirm the accuracy of the identification of the unit of blood, so Shirley dispensed with the second identity check and, after looking at the tag, she hung the unit. As before, the difference between the tag on the unit stating WN, 687116 and her patient, WM, 687115, was not apparent to her. As this unit began to be transfused, the patient's blood pressure fell even further and his temperature rose. Shirley noted that his urine was becoming bright red and the flow was slowing down, which is a sign of kidney failure. She notified

Bruce. The patient's breathing difficulties increased; Bruce decided to intubate him—place a tube in his trachea and attach the tube to a ventilator so the machine could breathe for him. Bruce became concerned that a transfusion reaction could be occurring and initiated a transfusion reaction work-up. In addition to collecting samples of blood and urine for laboratory analysis, this work-up involves checking for clerical errors.

The clerical check immediately determined that the patient WM, 687115, who had been identified as Sam Cohen by that time, had received two units of blood that were incompatible with his blood type. Sam was type O but had received two units of type A blood. Because blood type antigens cross-react with proteins in food and bacteria that we are all exposed to, adults have pre-existing antibodies to antigens that they lack. Thus, type O patients have anti-A antibodies that will immediately react with type A antigens, causing a transfusion reaction.

Sam went into shock. He developed blood-clotting problems associated with a transfusion reaction, an acute adult respiratory distress syndrome, and kidney failure. He was managed with life-support care for vital functions: fluids and diuretics to maintain kidney function, compatible blood products to treat the clotting problems, and medications to maintain his blood pressure. He was put on dialysis because his kidney function did not improve; he continued to need a ventilator to breathe. Sam did not recover from these complications; he died the next day without ever regaining consciousness. An internal hospital investigation of the incident identified multiple errors. Shirley Brown and Laura Peterson were allowed to resign in lieu of termination. Bruce Jones was allowed to continue his residency, but he never forgot the incident.

TRANSFUSION ISSUES

The preceding story is fiction, but it was inspired by actual events. The incident is typical in that there were multiple errors and multiple missed opportunities to have prevented the tragic outcome. Although many patients facing transfusion are most concerned about the risk of transmission of human immunodeficiency virus (HIV), few are concerned about receiving the incorrect blood through error. The risk of HIV transmission has been estimated at about 1/700,000, with the aggregate risk for transmission of any infectious disease of 1/34,000 (Schreiber, Busch, Kleinman, & Korelitz, 1996). These figures do not take into account the recent implementation of sophisticated molecular techniques to test for viral genetic material (DNA or RNA), which has reduced the infectious disease risk from transfusion even further, probably to less than 1/1,000,000 (Dodd, 2000).

The risk of receiving the wrong blood has been estimated at 1/14,000 units and the risk of getting an ABO incompatible unit is 1/41,000 (Linden, Wagner, Voytovich, & Sheehan, 2000). These risks of having the wrong blood transfused exceed the risks of transfusion transmission of all infectious diseases combined. The risk of a fatal reaction to an accidental incompatible blood transfusion has been estimated at 1/1,800,000 to 1/800,000 units (Linden et al., 2000; Mummert & Tourault, 1993; Sazama, 1990). That approximates or even exceeds the current risk of HIV transmission.

The magnitude of risk of being transfused with the wrong blood type is not unique to the United States. In the United Kingdom, the risk of getting the wrong unit of blood has been found to be 1/18,000 (McClelland & Phillips, 1994; Williamson et al., 1999). Of the adverse outcomes from blood transfusions in Britain over a 5-year period, 61% involved erroneous administration of the wrong unit, whereas only 2.6% involved transfusion-transmitted infections, such as HIV or hepatitis (Love et al., 2002). Even among transfusion-transmitted infections, error plays a role; 5 to 10% of the risk of such infections is attributed to laboratory error (Busch, Watanabe, & Smith, 2000). Transfusion transmission of HIV occurs because of errors such as transcribing the test results incorrectly or on another unit number (Courtois, Jullien, Chenais, Noel, & Pinon, 1992; Linden, 1994b; Salomão & Oliveira, 2000).

If a person receives an incorrect unit of blood, the odds are in favor of compatibility because preexisting antibodies related to cross-reacting antigens in food or bacteria occur only for the ABO antigen system. Patients who have not previously been pregnant or transfused are at risk only for ABO-related reactions. For other antigens, sensitization must occur through an initial exposure during pregnancy (from the baby's blood) or through transfusion. Once a patient is sensitized, however, subsequent transfusions must be matched for the additional antigens. For example, a patient who has developed antibody to the K antigen must receive blood tested and found negative for K and that does not react with the patient's blood during the crossmatch test.

In terms of ABO compatibility, a random unit of blood erroneously transfused to a random patient has, by chance alone, a statistical probability of 64% of being ABO compatible; that is, 64 times out of 100, the recipient's immune system would likely not react with the transfused red blood cells. Even patients unlucky enough to receive an ABO-incompatible unit may not experience a transfusion reaction, depending on the strength of their antibodies, the strength of the antigen, and quantity of blood transfused. Sam was unfortunate to have strong antibodies, was exposed to a strong antigen in the blood by mistake, and received a considerable volume of blood containing a foreign antigen.

There are multiple places in the transfusion process where errors can occur. A blood sample must be collected from the patient. The testing must be accurate and the unit properly labeled. The unit of blood must not be damaged by improper handling or by storing it at the wrong temperature such as placing it near a radiator, and it must be administered to the person for whom it was typed and crossmatched.

Errors In Sample Identification

The first step in the transfusion process is collecting the patient's blood sample for typing. Mislabeling of the sample after the blood was collected from the patient contributes to approximately 10% of cases of erroneous transfusion (Linden et al., 2000; Sazama, 1990). It has been found that 2.2% of patient identification wristbands contain errors and in 0.5% of these cases, the wristband contains another patient's information (Renner, Howanitz, & Bachner, 1993). Such errors are perpetuated on the samples of blood collected because the information on the label of the sample is based on the wristband. Proper labeling is critical. Blood samples that were incompletely labeled or labeled in the incorrect format were more than 40 times more likely to have been drawn from the wrong patient or labeled with incorrect information (Lumadue, Boyd, & Ness, 1997).

In Sam's case, the sample was correctly labeled, but because his name was not known at the time of initial treatment, fictitious initials were assigned. Because both the initials and numerical identifier were assigned sequentially, two patients with very similar identifiers were receiving care at the same time. This is an error waiting to happen. Laura Peterson's relative unfamiliarity of blood release procedures could have caused her to not differentiate the nearly identical identifiers on the blood units. The context in which Shirley Brown worked, the workload and dynamic conditions of the SICU, coupled with her concern for the patient, probably contributed to her not noticing the single alphabetic and single digit difference in the two patients' identifiers.

The existence of minimally different identifiers does not occur only in the emergency department; it also occurs when identifiers are assigned to newborns where a first name has not yet been given. This can be especially problematic in the case of multiple births as when Twin A Smith and Twin B Smith are assigned sequential medical record numbers. Marginally different identifiers also are assigned for patients who have the same last name and a similar or even identical first name, such as when father and son (senior and junior) are hospitalized simultaneously following a motor vehicle accident. This confusion not only may lead to incorrect blood transfusion, but other treatments may incorrectly be given, such as administering the wrong medications (Cohen, 1999; Lazarous, Pomeranz, & Corey, 1988).

Blood Bank Errors

Blood bank procedures are highly regimented; however, the procedures are effective only if they are followed. There are many steps in the procedures with the potential for an inappropriate action. One such step is testing. Blood bank testing errors account for about 15% of transfusion errors (Linden et al., 2000; Sazama, 1990). Testing presents many opportunities for error. In typing the sample, a blood bank staffer could take the wrong patient's sample from the test tube rack and use it for testing. In testing the sample, the typing chemicals could be added in the wrong order or not at all, so that a visible reaction would not occur. The reactions might not be interpreted correctly, giving rise to an incorrect determination of compatibility. There also is the opportunity for a clerical error, such as recording the results for one patient in the box on the results form designated for another patient. In Sam's case, Laura Peterson performed the testing correctly.

Blood bank errors also can occur at the point of releasing a unit of blood for transfusion. A common error is when blood removed from the refrigerator is tie-tagged with patient identifying information that is not correct for the specific unit of blood. Another possibility is that the blood given to the courier who comes to pick up blood for a particular patient is not the correct unit for that patient. Release of the wrong unit may occur in as many as 25 % of the cases of erroneous transfusion (Linden et al., 2000).

Returning to Sam's case, recall that Laura Peterson stored the crossmatched, ready-for-release units for WM, 687115 in the refrigerator next to those for WN, 687116, as was accepted practice. This practice contributed to the risk of Laura choosing the wrong unit. It is a systems factor that created an error-provoking situation. Even when the intent is to store blood of different types separately, errors occur. Units may not be placed in the correct designated section of a refrigerator. It has been reported that 0.12% of units are stored in the wrong section (for example, an A-positive unit placed in the "O-positive" section) and are liable to incorrect release if not checked very carefully (Shulman & Kent, 1991). The blood bank is not the only place where this occurs.

Confusing storage of blood frequently arises in the operating suite, where blood for different patients undergoing surgery that day is stored in the same refrigerator. If a patient develops complications and has an urgent need for blood, it is easy for the incorrect unit to be selected as the nurse hurries to get the blood to the patient as soon as possible (Linden, Paul, & Dressler, 1992; Sazama, 1990). Units of different blood types look similar and the only difference is the label. Correct reading of the label is critical, but one often tends to see what one expects to see, as illustrated by Sam's case.

The presence of a means of checking to confirm that the blood released is that for the specified patient does not mean it is effective. Computers have become common in blood banks to provide electronic rather than paper records of the release of units of blood. Those computers are able to double-check the ABO compatibility between the unit to be released and the patient's recorded blood type, keep track of the need for specially treated blood such as irradiated or white blood cell-reduced blood, and provide an alert if an inappropriate unit is intended for release. Such technological safeguards work only if they are used.

One disadvantage of technology, such as the computer, is that one may become dependent on it and lose proficiency with manual methods. To accommodate times when the computer is down, blood banks must have alternative manual methods to release units; however, when the computer is down (or not used), staff may be even more prone to error than if the computer were not in use at all. This is what happened to Laura Peterson as she intended to save time. Thus, it can be seen that a combination of system factors predisposed Laura to make the error of choosing the wrong unit and failing to notice she had done so: She was assigned to perform unfamiliar tasks in the blood bank, her workload was high causing her to rush, her work was interrupted, units of different blood types were next to each other in the refrigerator, and the computer checking was cumbersome to use.

A final opportunity to detect the release of the wrong blood for a patient occurs at the bedside when the nurse verifies correspondence of the patient's identification information with the information on the unit. Often, as illustrated by Sam's case, a variety of circumstances preclude this opportunity for detection.

Identification Errors

Administration of blood to the incorrect recipient constitutes the largest single human error in the transfusion system, accounting for about 40% of cases (Linden et al., 2000; Sazama, 1990; Taswell, Galbreath, & Harmsen, 1994; Tissier, Le Pennec, Hergon, & Rouger, 1996). Figure 2.1 illustrates a nurse administering a unit of blood. In many cases, the person administering the blood (usually a nurse) assumes that the blood received is for a patient for whom blood is expected and administers it without adequately verifying identification. The nurse may glance at the wristband, without truly reading it, or may be confident of the patient's identity and not check it at all; however, the nurse could read the wristband closely but, because of nearly identical identifying information, be unable to discriminate the patient's identity between it and the unit tag. In most hospitals, the comparison of the name and identification number on the unit tag with the information on the patient's wristband is performed manually by two people, with one reading the information verbally to the other. Other hospitals use automated handheld barcode readers or other devices designed to assist in identification (Jensen & Crosson, 1996; Langeberg, Berg, Novak, & Sandler, 1999; Wenz & Burns, 1991).

In approximately 15% of erroneous transfusions, the blood bank issues the wrong unit; proper identification procedures at the bedside could detect the

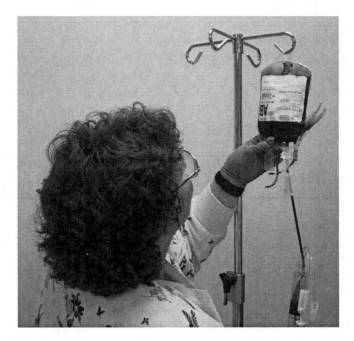

FIG. 2.1.   A nurse administers a unit of blood.

error, but that does not occur (Linden et al., 2000). That was the case in our story—nurse Shirley Brown could have detected that the wrong unit was issued, but because she was rushed and was misled by the similar identifiers, just as Laura Peterson had been, and no one was available to confirm the identification, the difference was not detected. Identical or similar names often figure prominently in cases of blood misadministration (Linden et al., 2000; Sazama, 1990). This can occur if staff are busy, preoccupied with other matters, or overly confident that they know the patient and assume that the blood that arrives is for that patient, as illustrated in Sam's case.

Failure To Recognize An Adverse Event

Nurse Shirley Brown detected signs that were out of the norm of those expected for the conditions of the case (the decrease in blood pressure, fever, and pink urine). She was busy and not thinking about the possibility of a transfusion reaction because such reactions are rare; she did not interpret the signs as indicating an impending dire situation and did not report them in a timely fashion to the physician on duty. When she did report the signs, the resident physician initially attributed them to the patient's condition and did not suspect a transfusion reaction even though the signs the patient exhibited are cardinal signs of such a reaction. This often occurs in very ill patients, for whom the clinical picture may be complex and who may exhibit signs for reasons related to the underlying medical condition, such as trauma. Nonetheless, if there is any doubt, a transfusion reaction work-up should be performed to rule out that possibility; however, as in this case, physicians may be reluctant to delay treatment. Cost also can be a disincentive.

The index of suspicion for a transfusion reaction often is low for patients receiving their own (autologous) blood. The physician assumes that the blood must be compatible without considering the possibility of an administration error. Erroneous administrations do occur with supposedly autologous blood whereby such blood is administered to another patient in the same room or is given to a patient with a similar name (Goldman, Rémy-Prince, Trépanier, & Décary, 1997; Linden, 1994a; Mackey & Lipton, 1995). Such errors pose not only the risk of transfusion reaction, but also the risk of transmission of infectious diseases, because autologous blood for a patient's own use may be collected from patients who carry infectious diseases. The blood may not be tested or may be used even if known positive on infectious disease testing, as it will be used only for that patient. Reinfusing a patient's own blood shortly after it was recovered during surgery could pose a risk of air entering the patient's circulatory system because the blood recovery device collects air along with the blood (Linden, Kaplan, & Murphy, 1997). This air could cause a fatal cardiac arrest.

In Sam's case, both residents may have had insufficient training in recognizing transfusion reactions, had not previously observed such a reaction, and did not apply their classroom training to the real world. They may have assumed that blood transfusion is a simple process and it did not occur to them that, in dealing with very serious injuries, something could go wrong with the transfusion. Because they did not expect a transfusion reaction, they did not request the work-up, but, seeking to provide good care to the patient, ordered another unit that unfortunately followed the same pattern of error. When appropriate therapy was initiated, it was too late to save the patient.

CONCLUSION

Transfusion errors occur with alarming frequency. The causes of errors are multifactored; there are multiple points in the transfusion process at which the error can be detected and prevented. The processes and procedures often are overly complex and confusing and, as such, predispose to error. In Sam's case, the similar identifiers made it difficult for nursing staff and laboratory staff to discern the differences between him and another patient. Storage of different units next to each other in a refrigerator likewise can predispose to confusion and error. The lack of experience with transfusion reactions and the lack of expectation for such an event led both the nurses and physicians initially to not recognize what was occurring.

The transfusion process requires cooperation between sample collection staff, the blood bank, and staff in patient care areas. A mistake at any point may lead to the patient receiving the incorrect blood. Patient or sample identification errors, occurring either at the time of collection of the blood sample or at the time of transfusion, are the most common problem. The blood bank, however, may perform testing incorrectly or issue the incorrect unit. Distraction, a heavy workload, or fatigue can contribute to the possibility that staff may inappropriately perform familiar procedures.

Identification procedures that result in similar identifiers make the task of distinguishing different patients or blood units more challenging and error prone. In other cases, cumbersome procedures that require manual steps without the assistance of an automated device or computer place a burden on staff to recognize subtle differences. An opportunity for early intervention may be missed if the signs of a reaction are not recognized when incompatible blood is erroneously given. The case presented illustrates some of the types of events that can contribute to a preventable adverse outcome. Analysis of errors to determine contributing system factors can lead to the adjustment of the way things are done to reduce or avoid situations that predispose staff to make mistakes.

REFERENCES

Busch, M. P., Watanabe, K. K., Smith, J. W., Hermansen, S. W., & Thomson, R. A. (2000). False-negative testing errors in routine virus marker screening of blood donors. The Retrovirus Epidemiology Donor Study. *Transfusion, 40,* 585–589.

Cohen, M. R. (Ed.). (1999). *Medication errors.* Washington, DC: American Pharmaceutical Association.

Courtois, F., Jullien, A. M., Chenais, F., Noel, L., & Pinon, F. (1992). Transfusion of HIV by transfusion of HIV-screened blood: The value of a national register. The recipients' study group of the French Society of Blood Transfusion. *Transfusion Medicine, 2,* 51–55.

Dodd, R. (2000). Germs, gels and genomes: A personal recollection of 30 years in blood safety testing. In S. Stramer (Ed.), *Blood safety in the new millennium* (pp. 97–122). Bethesda, MD: American Association of Blood Banks.

Goldman, M., Rémy-Prince, S., Trépanier, A., & Décary, F. (1997). Autologous donation error rates in Canada. *Transfusion, 37,* 523–527.

Jensen, N. J., & Crosson, J. T. (1996). An automated system for bedside verification of the match between patient identification and blood group identification. *Transfusion, 36,* 216–221.

Langeberg, A. F., Berg, M., Novak, S. C., & Sandler, S. G. (1999). Evaluation of the Immucor I-TRAC System for positive patient, blood sample and blood unit identification [abstract]. *Transfusion, 39,* 25S.

Lazarous, J., Pomeranz, B. H., & Corey, P. N. (1988). Incidence of adverse drug reactions in hospitalized patients: a meta-analysis of prospective studies. *Journal of the American Medical Association, 279,* 1200–1205.

Linden, J. V. (1994a). Autologous blood errors and incidents [abstract]. *Transfusion, 34,* 28S.

Linden, J. V. (1994b). Error contributes to the risk of transmissible disease [letter]. *Transfusion, 34,* 1016.

Linden, J. V., Kaplan, H. S., & Murphy, M. T. (1997). Fatal air embolism due to perioperative blood recovery. *Anesthesia and Analgesia, 84,* 422–426.

Linden, J. V., Paul, B., & Dressler, K. P. (1992). A report of 104 transfusion errors in New York State. *Transfusion, 32,* 601–606.

Linden, J. V., Wagner, K., Voytovich, A. E., & Sheehan, J. (2000). Transfusion errors in New York State: An analysis of 10 years' experience. *Transfusion, 40,* 1207–1213.

Love, E., Asher, D., Atterbury, C. L. J., Chapman, C., Cohen, H., Jones, H., Norfolk, D. R., Revill, J., Soldan, K., Todd, A., & Williamson, L. M. (2002). *The serious hazards of transfusion.* Annual Report, 2000–2001, Royal College of Pathologists, Manchester, UK.

Lumadue, J. A., Boyd, J. S., & Ness, P. M. (1997). Adherence to a strict specimen-labeling policy decreases the incidence of erroneous blood grouping of blood bank specimens. *Transfusion, 37,* 1169–1172.

Mackey, J., & Lipton, K. S. (1995). AABB position on testing of autologous units. *Association Bulletin, 95-4.* Bethesda, MD: American Association of Blood Banks.

McClelland, D. B. L., & Phillips, P. (1994). Errors in blood transfusion in Britain: survey of hospital haematology departments. *British Medical Journal, 308,* 1205–1206.

Mummert, T. B., & Tourault, M. A. (1993). Review of transfusion related fatalities: many preventable. *Hospital Scanner, 11,* 1–3.

Renner, S. W., Howanitz, P. J., & Bachner, P. (1993). Wristband identification error reporting in 712 hospitals. *Archives of Pathology and Laboratory Medicine, 117,* 573–577.

Salomão, R., & Oliveira, J. S. F. (2000). Passive transfer of HIV-1 antibodies and absence of HIV infection after the transfusion of HIV-1 seropositive red cells [letter]. *Transfusion, 40,* 252–253.

Sazama, K. (1990). Reports of 355 transfusion-associated deaths: 1976 through 1985. *Transfusion, 30,* 583–590.

Schreiber, G. B., Busch, M. P., Kleinman, S. H., & Korelitz, J. J. (1996). The risk of transfusion-transmitted viral infection. *New England Journal of Medicine, 334,* 1685–1690.

Shulman, I. A., & Kent, D. (1991). Unit placement errors: A potential risk factor for ABO and Rh incompatible blood transfusions. *Laboratory Medicine, 22,* 194–196.

Taswell, H. F., Galbreath, J. L., & Harmsen, W. S. (1994). Errors in transfusion medicine. Detection, analysis, frequency, and prevention. *Archives of Pathology and Laboratory Medicine, 118,* 405–410.

Tissier, A. M., Le Pennec, P. Y., Hergon, E., & Rouger, P. (1996). Immunohemolytic transfusion reactions. IV. Analysis, risks, and prevention (English abstract). *Transfusion Clinique et Biologique, 3,* 167–180.

Wenz, B., & Burns, E. R. (1991). Improvement in transfusion safety using a new blood unit and patient identification system as part of a safe transfusion practice. *Transfusion, 31,* 401–403.

Williamson, L. M., Lowe, S., Love, E., Cohen, H., Soldan, K., McClelland, D. B. L., Norfolk, D. R., Revill, J., Barbara, J. A. J., Birrell, D., & Todd, A. (1999). *The serious hazards of transfusion. Annual Report, 1997–1998.* Manchester, UK: Royal College of Pathologists.

3 Stopping Bad Things From Happening to Good People in Shock Trauma Centers

Colin F. Mackenzie
Yan Xiao
University of Maryland School of Medicine

SHOCK TRAUMA CENTER
MEDICAL STUDENT, BEN JOHNSON

Ben Johnson was a final-year medical student. He was very excited at the prospect of working in the trauma center because this would be the first time he would function like a real doctor. It was his first night on call. Everyone was busy in the operating room so he was relieved that there had been no new patients admitted. At 10:15 p.m. there was a loud ring on the emergency phone. Ben's heart raced. Jennifer Kung, a trauma nurse, answered the phone and was getting a report from the paramedics at the injury scene. Jennifer wrote several abbreviated items of summary information on a board where incoming cases are posted for all to see. Ben noticed on the board that the incoming patient was a pedestrian struck by a car. Expected time of arrival was 5 minutes. Jennifer did not know the patient's name. Magically to Ben, nurses, physicians, and technicians appeared from the operating room area, from the group of previously laughing and joking nurses around the coffeemaker, and from the entrance doors to the resuscitation area.

Ben knew the surgical staff members. Stuart Kennerley was a second-year resident physician who had graduated from medical school just over 2 years earlier and had about a year of on-the-job training. Although Ben did not know it, Stuart had several other patients who were admitted to the trauma center earlier on his mind; he also had not slept for more than 2 hours without interruption over the past 36 hours. Stuart came to the resuscitation area from the operating

27

room where he was helping the surgical attending physician and another surgical resident physician with an operation on a patient admitted earlier. Stuart knew they needed help performing the surgery and wanted to assist them, but he was sent to admit the new patient. He called Ben over, asking him to be in charge of the incoming patient admission: "We don't have a lot of information on this patient, but it doesn't appear to be a critical injury." Ben did not know all of the people who would be working on the new patient. He recognized the two trauma nurses, but did not know much about two other people who came to assist in this patient's admission. "They must be anesthesiologists," Ben thought.

When paramedics brought the patient in, Ben realized that he was severely injured. The paramedics reported that the patient had been struck by a fast-moving car, causing head injuries and a broken leg. While at the injury scene, the paramedics started cardiopulmonary resuscitation; they could not put in an intravenous line to supply fluids to the patient because he was an intravenous drug abuser and had "used up" his veins for his drug habit. Ben was surprised that those critical items of information were not mentioned before the patient's arrival, nor were they listed with the summary information on the posting board.

Stuart felt overwhelmed because the patient's injuries were much more serious than he had expected, so Ben, given his level of training, really could not be fully in charge of him. Stuart wished that he had more time to organize everyone and get more help, including a neurosurgeon to examine any potential neurological injuries to the patient's head and neck. This was the first time Ben had worked with the anesthesiologists who were giving oxygen and ventilating the lungs of the patient referred to as John Doe because he had no identification. While that was being done, Ben and Stuart were trying to put in an intravenous line to prepare John Doe for possible placement of a tube into the chest to drain blood that might accumulate after the injury.

As Ben was trying to put in an intravenous line, he could not hear instructions from Stuart because of the noise from all of the activity around the patient. When the blood pressure and other vital signs monitors were connected to the semi-conscious, moaning John Doe, several loud alarms went off because he was struggling and had to be restrained, all of which interfered with the functioning of the monitors. The neurosurgeon was paged; until she arrived and conducted the neurological examination, the team had to wait. Only after the neurosurgeon's examination could the patient be anesthetized. Ben was eager for that to happen so he would not have to hold down the struggling patient and could proceed with his plan. Bob Koone, the anesthesiologist, was concerned about the struggling John Doe, who ran the risk of injuring himself and the people around him. He was receiving adequate oxygen via a facemask, but Bob knew his condition could deteriorate soon without the life-saving interventions. Those inter-

ventions were needed immediately, but first the patient had to be anesthetized. Did the surgery people have a plan, he wondered?

Bob was glad that he had come with an experienced resident anesthesiologist, George Blank. Where is the neurosurgeon, they wondered? When the neurosurgeon finally responded, 7 minutes after John Doe's arrival, it seemed that all the alarms were sounding from his monitors as well as the alarms from monitors connected to patients in nearby treatment bays. The neurological examination was brief, and found serious injuries to the brain. Rapid diagnostic procedures and emergency interventions were needed. John Doe was anesthetized. Bob, the anesthesiologist, asked George, the resident, to pass a breathing tube into John Doe's windpipe that would be attached to a device that would breathe for him. This would allow Bob time to prepare the next steps in treating John Doe.

George found it difficult to see the structures inside the mouth to insert the breathing tube because John Doe's throat was bloody from his injuries. The first two passes of the tube mistakenly went into the esophagus (connecting the mouth to the stomach) instead of the trachea (connecting the mouth to the lungs). On the third pass, George felt he inserted the tube into the trachea. Bob watched with some anxiety and waited for some indication from the monitors confirming that the tube was in the patient's trachea. A high-pitched alarm was sounding that George wanted to silence, but he could not reach the patient monitors to reset them. "One of the surgeons is listening to the chest to determine if the breathing tube actually is in the trachea," thought Bob, the anesthesiologist, as he saw Ben placing a stethoscope on the chest. The sounds from the patient's chest could provide an early indication of where the breathing tube was placed; however, this method is not failure-proof, and listening to the chest requires training. Using a stethoscope, one should hear equal breath sounds on both sides of the chest and no breath sounds in the stomach if the breathing tube is properly placed.

George did not realize that Ben was a medical student who was not qualified to perform the important task of verifying breathing tube placement. When a misplaced tube is uncorrected, the patient's lungs do not receive oxygen; a patient will suffer brain damage and die if no oxygen is received for 5 minutes. Ben listened to the patient's chest. George, the anesthesiologist resident, asked Ben: "Did you hear breath sounds?" Ben nodded his head. Then Ben listened to the stomach, although not sure what he was supposed to hear. He heard sounds again there. He said, "It's also going in here too." No one seemed to hear that comment, however. Bob, the anesthesiologist, because of the noise from the alarms and from laughter and chatting in an adjacent area, did not hear what Ben said about the breathing sound from the patient's stomach.

The gold standard of confirming the placement of the breathing tube calls for the monitoring of the patient's exhaled carbon dioxide. When the breathing tube is properly placed, the carbon dioxide from the patient's lungs flows through the breathing tube and can be measured. When no carbon dioxide is detected from the breathing tube, one can be certain that the breathing tube is misplaced. The positioning of the breathing equipment set-up would not allow Bob or George to easily connect the breathing tube to a carbon dioxide monitor. They trusted Ben's judgment and proceeded to tape the breathing tube in position, as they do after successful placement.

Stuart, the second-year surgical resident physician, had assumed that the breathing tube was properly placed and had started cutting into the patient's chest to place the chest tube to drain the blood. The alarm sounded from the pulse oximeter, a monitor measuring the oxygen concentration in the patient's blood by means of sensor clipped on the patient's finger. The alarm suggested that John Doe was not receiving adequate oxygen. Bob looked at the reading on the pulse oximeter. It displayed 50%, and then 40%, with a normal reading being above 95% and close to 100%. This was too low; perhaps the reading should not be trusted because the patient was struggling and moving about which could have caused misplacement of the finger sensor, Bob reasoned. He checked other monitors and noticed that the automated blood pressure monitor was attempting to obtain a measurement, but for some reason had not succeeded in the last several minutes.

Bob and George waited, becoming anxious because they did not know John Doe's status. They did not communicate their concerns to other team members, such as Stuart and Ben, who were occupied with placing the drain in the patient's chest. Finally, John Doe's blood pressure and pulse oximeter monitors displayed a set of readings that were very abnormal. By this time Bob suspected that the breathing tube was not placed properly and patient had not been receiving oxygen. Bob asked George to reconfigure the breathing circuitry so the exhaled carbon dioxide could be monitored. There was no carbon dioxide detected in the breathing tube. It was now quite clear that the breathing tube had been misplaced into the esophagus. The patient had been without oxygen for 6 minutes! If he were not to die from the injuries from the motor vehicle crash, he surely would die from the prolonged undetected misplacement of the breathing tube.

CHALLENGES IN TRAUMA CARE

This story consists of several actual occurrences rolled into one fictional case that illustrates the unique set of challenges physicians and nurses face working in a trauma center. The workload can vary tremendously during one shift because the care providers do not know when and how many patients will arrive at any time. They often must act quickly with little information to save the patient's life.

Physicians and nurses who do not know each other and have not worked together previously are thrust together to perform procedures that require practiced coordination of efforts. These challenging activities to provide care to people in the most acute states of trauma occur in a physical environment that typically is crowded, cramped, and seemingly characterized by a controlled chaos. The optimal care of an injured victim at a trauma center depends on many components. Even with the best health care technology and highly trained physicians and nurses, medical errors can still occur, often provoked by conditions of systems factors in the context in which care is provided.

Information and Communications

There are circumstances that make management of trauma patients unlike any other medical emergency. When treating trauma patients, the physicians and nurses often have very little information and no medical history for the patients. In the story, Jennifer Kung received only a few pieces of information about John Doe when she spoke to the paramedic in the field. Ben was unaware that no intravenous access had been obtained because John Doe was a drug abuser. Stuart had no idea that John Doe was in critical condition from the information he saw on the posting board.

Injured patients coming to a trauma center may be unconscious and unable to remember past medical histories and allergies, or recall the details of what had just happened. The precipitating event, such as a motor vehicle crash, usually is unexpected, life threatening, and may result in impaired consciousness or amnesia. As a result of these circumstances, the receiving medical team at a trauma center has very little idea of the site or extent of a patient's injury. The event often happens when family or friends are not with the patient or they also are injured in the same incident. Thus, typically for trauma patients, there is a lack of information about medications being taken or previous surgeries (Mackenzie & Lippert, 1999).

The first notification of an impending patient admission occurs via a call on the radio connection between paramedics located at the injury scene and the on-call trauma surgeon in the trauma center. In the story, the trauma surgeon was occupied in the operating room, so the call was taken by a trauma nurse, Jennifer Kung. The summary information from this communication from the field paramedics is written on a board (Fig. 3.1). Information posted on the board notifies the trauma team members so they can prepare an admitting trauma bay.

That bay is one of a number of nearly identical areas with equipment and an examining table; each bay can be separated from the others by movable curtains.

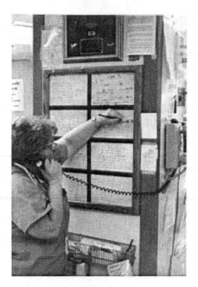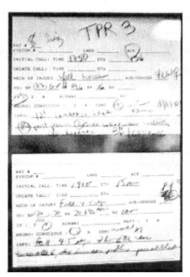

FIG. 3.1.   The Doe Board, a display board that stores and displays incoming patient information and location of admitted patients.

Because John Doe's status deteriorated rapidly and required cardiopulmonary resuscitation, the paramedics did not have time to communicate an update on his status. Without that information, the trauma team did not anticipate, hence did not prepare for, admitting a critically ill patient.

As illustrated by the story, because John Doe was unconscious and alone, no information was available about his medical history, and very little information was provided about how his injuries occurred and the treatment at the injury scene. As in this case, the paramedics can be too busy to pass on information in a timely manner without interrupting patient care procedures. There is no standardized way for the paramedics to update the trauma centers on the status of possible admission of a trauma patient. Variations in what is reported can lead to gaps in information. As a result, not only is there a lack of information about the trauma patient, there also is a lack of communication conveying what information is available. Observations at the injury scene are communicated only 75% of the time; additional information is helpful in 52% of cases (Brown & Warwick, 2001).

Efficient flow of information about patients and their injuries and the quality of the information can make a difference to those who need to prepare to take care of the patients. When the patient is a child, pediatric-sized equipment is prepared; if the patient is unconscious, the neurosurgeon is called. In the story, because Ben and Stuart were unprepared to receive such a critically injured patient, they did not call the neurosurgeon early. Bob, the anesthesiologist, had to wait, struggling to restrain John Doe, until the neurosurgeon examined him. After that, he could anesthetize him. The surgical team that had to wait until John Doe was anesthetized could start operating on his chest to drain the blood. Thus, the lack of information about the patient's condition restricted the planning opportunities and prolonged the time necessary to start emergency interventions.

Problems with the flow of information can occur when the description of the patient and injury is verbally relayed because misunderstandings may occur. If the first communication from the field describes a patient with a gunshot wound to the head arriving in 3 minutes as an emergency, the trauma team members stop whatever they are doing and move quickly to the patient arrival and resuscitation area. If that patient arrives later or does not have a gunshot wound, then the performance of the care providers can be affected. Such lack of adequate communication is a major contributor to medical errors (Donchin et al., 1995). Indeed, physicians and nurses often view lack of communication within organizations and teams as the leading source of uncertainties in trauma care (Xiao, 1997).

If the age of the patient is not clearly conveyed to the trauma center by the prehospital care provider, then mismatches between preparation and patient can occur, such as a 2-year-old patient arriving to a trauma team that is prepared only for an adult. Errors can occur when the care providers are stressed by spending precious time obtaining pediatric equipment or when attempting to save precious time by adapting adult equipment to fit a pediatric patient. Examples of communication issues include not only omissions in verbal reports and lack of needed details, but also delays and illegible handwriting notations. When the correct information about the patient and his or her injuries is communicated from the scene to the trauma center, an efficient system distributes that information to the trauma team and appropriate procedures are instituted. In the story, the nature of John Doe's injuries was not adequately conveyed by the paramedics to the people at the trauma center because they were performing cardiopulmonary resuscitation and could not take time away from patient care to update their earlier communication.

The distribution of information inside the trauma center can be hampered by the technology involved. For example, dead spots exist in the trauma center where the pagers do not function due to radio signal transmission not being available. Because of this, some key members of the trauma team may not receive paging messages. This is especially important when there is a short interval between the time of the call from the field-care provider paramedic and the estimated time of arrival at the trauma center. The trauma team members may be doing other tasks in the intensive care unit or operating room, or catching up on lost sleep in the basement sleep quarters, and have to make arrangements to get to the trauma unit. For example, Stuart, who is chronically sleep-deprived because of his workload, takes any opportunity to catch up on sleep whenever possible. It is important for patient safety that Stuart and all care providers are well rested because fatigue is a significant factor affecting vigilance and performance in the operating room (Weinger & Englund, 1990).

With a long interval between the first call from the field and patient arrival, or multiple consecutive patient admissions, the trauma team member is likely to learn about the next patient admission from colleagues or team members also on call. Lack of information about patient injuries or age is particularly challenging because it can make designation of personnel difficult. Physicians and nurses must make decisions on how to deploy their resources, especially when they have multiple tasks demanding their attention in different parts of the hospital— conditions that stress them to the extreme.

Composition and Preparation of Trauma Teams

Physicians and nurses are assigned in an ad hoc manner for each incoming trauma patient; this is done to some extent to accommodate physician training. The regular members of the team (attending physicians and nurses) become accustomed to the constant change of faces among the physicians in training who often stay for 1 or 2 months at a time. In the story, the anesthesiologists did not challenge a medical student's comment about the patient status and ability to hear breath sounds in the chest. To the anesthesiologists, the student was just another new member of the team and wore no identification of the fact that he was a student and not a qualified doctor. Without a formal organization, the ad hoc trauma team put the inexperienced student in the position of a decision maker where he clearly was inadequately trained. Furthermore, the lack of information about the incoming patient had rendered the team unprepared. Unlike aviation, where teams meet before a scheduled flight, the trauma team did not meet before John Doe arrived. The team had to wait for the neurosurgeon, because this consultant usually is not present for trauma patient admissions, but is called only for a special consult when needed.

Trauma patient diagnoses are refined by means of investigations, such as radiography (x-rays) and portable ultrasound scanning devices (similar to the devices used to observe babies in the womb) that detect blood in the abdomen noninvasively, and by the findings from the laboratory blood tests. The priorities for the initial assessment and management are outlined as guidelines developed by the American College of Surgeons. These Advanced Trauma Life Support (ATLS) Guidelines are a prototypical approach to provide a best-practice model for the trauma team that works in a high-risk environment where tasks need to be carried out under severe time pressures with many stressors including noise and uncertainty. Often nonroutine decisions have to be made with imperfect information, and there may be no correct answer.

The ATLS Guidelines only provide a framework for management decisions; they do not consider the cultural, legal, and administrative practices in place at a given trauma center. In the story, the attending surgeon who was Ben's supervisor was in the operating room dealing with an emergency that had arisen in one of the trauma patients admitted earlier in the day. For medical, legal, and patient billing purposes, it is necessary that the attending surgeon be in the operating room for this key portion of the case. Because of this, he was not able to help when the John Doe admission occurred. The culture of the trauma center training was that Ben, as the medical student, had to stand by his decisions, although he would normally consult his attending surgeon when they had both completed interventions for their current emergency situations.

Teams in the domain of trauma patient resuscitation have characteristics that can result in lack of coordination in emergencies. Team members are trained differently (for example, surgery and anesthesiology), so the surgeon does not always understand the issues associated with decision making of the anesthesiologist and vice versa. Teams including those that perform surgical procedures may include personnel in training and their supervisors. Because trainees in an ad hoc trauma team may not be identified clearly as students and their supervisor may be occupied in another location, as was the case with Ben Johnson, inappropriate responsibility may be given to a person who is not adequately trained to perform the task.

Team composition changes from case to case because the work schedules of each of the surgeons, anesthesiologists, and nurses rotate differently. For example, the surgeon who first admits a patient may not operate on the patient; rather, the orthopedist consultant may operate with the anesthesiologist. These differing schedules can easily lead to problems in communication such that important information does not get passed on. In many of the teams, there is no time for a formal hand-over process of briefing the next care provider on the condition and other factors regarding the patient because of urgent needs for their skills elsewhere in the emergency department. Resuscitation teams, not having gone through teamwork training, consider the roles and job specifications for each team member largely on the basis of tradition. This means that, depending on the members of any given ad hoc team, there may be gaps in expertise or inappropriate focus on one aspect of management to the detriment of overall care of the emergency trauma patient.

Physical Working Environment

In the trauma center patient admitting area, there is considerable activity and noise, making hearing especially difficult. Admitting a patient to the trauma

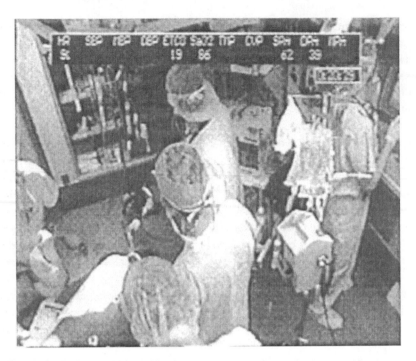

FIG. 3.2.   Video image of trauma patient resuscitation. This patient had a flail chest and major intra-abdominal bleeding. Vital signs show heart rate on extreme left. End-tidal CO_2, O_2 saturation, and noninvasive blood pressure shown on the right side of overlay.

center takes place in a large room divided into bays enclosed by curtains and movable dividers; there is no separate room for each patient with walls that dampen some of the noise. When Ben listens to John Doe's belly and hears air entering the stomach, his comment "and it's going in here, too" is drowned out by conversations and laughter from the vacant adjacent resuscitation bay where some technicians and staff are discussing last night's ball game. Nontask-related communications and patient monitor alarms, the majority of which are false alarms, greatly increase the likelihood of ineffective verbal communication.

In each of the trauma center bays, the workspace layout is a compromise between what space is available in a 13′ by 12′ (4 meters by 3.6 meters) area to devote solely to one task, and what space is occupied by the patient and the trauma team members (Fig. 3.2). There is no systematic analysis that can determine a safe design of the workplace for all emergency procedures. The major requirement for the space is flexibility to allow use in all contingencies. As a result, the layout is not ideal for many tasks—for example, emergency airway management. Notice the haphazard nature of equipment placement in Fig. 3.2.

The trauma team, which may number six or more persons with expertise in nursing, anesthesiology, and surgery, all congregate in the space around the gurney on which the patient is placed when the field-care providers arrive in the trauma center patient admitting area. Equipment for monitoring vital signs and intravenous fluids surround the team—the workplace often is cluttered (Harper, Mackenzie, & Norman, 1995).

At the head of the bed, the anesthesiology team stands ready to manage the airway and to assist the surgical and nursing team with intravenous access. At the right shoulder, a trauma nurse is prepared to take vital signs on admission and draw a blood sample for laboratory tests. At the foot of the patient and on the left side stands the surgical team, with the surgical team leader standing beside the area of the patient's left chest. Resuscitation of the patient is guided by corrections of abnormalities in vital signs such as blood pressure and heart rate, and maintaining other vital functions, including airway patency, breathing, and circulation. Abnormal vital signs are normalized by intravenous fluid, blood, and medication administration.

Time is a critical factor in patient survival; 80% of trauma deaths occur in the first 4 hours after injury (Brown, 1987). Time pressure also compounds with the uncertainty, as the resuscitation team may not have the luxury of waiting for extensive patient monitoring information but may have to act with what is available (Xiao et al., 1996). The frequency of false patient monitor alarms, and the unreliability of data displayed by physiologic monitors due to patient movement and other interferences with the measurement connection to the patient, increases the uncertainty in confirming correct placement of the airway tube. Bob, the anesthesiologist in the story, rationalized the low pulse oximeter reading as being due to finger sensor misplacement, rather than a true reading, because so often this was the cause of such a low value. In addition, because the equipment was set up to be ready for mechanical ventilation, the carbon-dioxide analyzer was connected in the ventilator, not the hand-squeezed ventilating device used by Ben Johnson's teammates.

CONCLUSION

The trauma unit is perhaps the most intense and stressful of any unit in a hospital. Time is of critical importance—a few minutes can make the difference between life and death. Despite the sometimes superhuman efforts by the trauma unit staff, errors occur such as the one in the story. The typical response to an adverse outcome is to hold the care provider responsible. As the story of Ben Johnson illustrates, multiple factors affected several of the care providers, culminating in the adverse event. To reduce the likelihood of such an event happening again, it is necessary to analyze the situation that gave rise to the event to determine error-provoking factors. For example, systems factors such as noise in the work environment can impair critically important communications. Had Ben Johnson's comment "and it's going on here, too" been heard, the remaining chain of events might never have occurred.

Despite the commonly held belief that technology is the answer to many problems in health care, that it is far superior to the human, dependence on technology to the exclusion of clinical examination of the patient led to the experienced anesthesiology care providers allowing a medical student, rather than themselves, listen to the patient's chest. The anesthesiology team had such faith in technology that abnormally low oxygen values displayed on the monitor were considered merely artifacts of the activity of John Doe. That faith in technology was so great that the low reading from the oxygen monitor was not checked against the monitor value for the amount of exhaled CO_2. Had their faith in technology not been so great and the other value checked, the inappropriate placement of the breathing tube would have been detected shortly after insertion.

Although supervision of fatigued and inexperienced care providers not only is necessary for patient safety through the effective coordination of activities, supervision also is necessary in the training of medical students as emerging physicians. Experienced personnel circumvent problems by obtaining information from multiple sources. They know most if not all members of an ad hoc team and are more familiar with available options, hence are able to make a rapid assessment of the situation and plan ahead for contingencies.

Uncertainty during initial emergency trauma patient management leads to decision making with incomplete or inaccurate information, so that errors and task omissions occur with a higher frequency than in elective management. Because the condition of the trauma patient dynamically changes at a rapid rate, information not regularly updated may be incorrect or misleading and lead to inappropriate treatment. Workload varies in emergency management, affecting staff scheduling and other administrative issues such as resupply, which can impact patient safety.

Thus, an adverse outcome that might be attributed to a human error is actually a Gordian knot of contributing factors, each of which may be necessary but none sufficient to cause the incident. The reduction of error and the concomitant enhancement of patient safety lies in identifying and addressing those factors.

ACKNOWLEDGMENT

Funded in part by the Agency for Health Care Research & Quality, Grant #5U18HS11279-02, and by the Department of Anesthesiology, University of Maryland School of Medicine (CFM Sabbatical).

REFERENCES

Brown, D. L. (1987). Trauma management: The anesthesiologist's role. *International Anesthesiology Clinics, 25,* 1–18.

Brown, R., & Warwick, J. (2001). Blue calls—time for a change? *Emergency Medicine Journal, 18*(4), 289–92.

Donchin, Y., Gopher, D., Olin, M., Badihi, Y., Biesky, M., Sprung, C. L., Pizov, R., & Cotev, S. (1995). A look into the nature and causes of human errors in the intensive care unit. *Critical Care Medicine, 23*(2), 294–300.

Harper, B. D., Mackenzie, C. F., & Norman, K. L. (1995). *Quantitative measures in the ergonomic examination of the trauma resuscitation units anesthesia workspace.* Proceedings of Human Factors and Ergonomics Society 39th Annual Meeting (pp. 723–727). Santa Monica, CA: Human Factors and Ergonomics Society.

Mackenzie, C. F., & Lippert, F. K. (1999). Emergency department management of trauma. *Anesthesiology Clinics of North America, 17,* 45–61.

Weinger, M. B., & Englund, C. E. (1990). Ergonomic and human factors affecting anesthetic vigilance and monitoring performance in the operating room environment. *Anesthesiology, 73,* 995–1021.

Xiao, Y. (1997). *Uncertainty in trauma patient resuscitation.* Proceedings of Human Factors and Ergonomics Society 41st Annual Meeting (pp 168–171). Santa Monica, CA: Human Factors and Ergonomics Society.

Xiao, Y., Hunter, W., Mackenzie, C. F., Jeffery, N. J., Horst, R. L., & LOTAS Group. (1996). Task complexity in emergency medical care and its implications for team coordination. *Human Factors, 38,* 636–645.

4 Misadventures in General Surgery

Ramon Berguer
University of California, Davis
Veterans Administration Northern California
Health Care System

Every surgeon knows what it means to have a bad day. In a few hours, and often despite the best efforts of those involved, events occur that can seriously injure a patient and destroy a surgeon's career. In cases like these, everyone involved loses. Are these occurrences part and parcel of treating surgical illness? Are they modern medicine at its worst?

SURGEON, ROBERT SMITH, M.D.

For Dr. Robert Smith, 35, the road to becoming a surgeon had been a long one. Four years of medical school were followed by 6 years of surgical training and an appointment as a surgeon and a junior faculty member at a leading university medical center. One weekend in October, Dr. Smith was on call, meaning that from Friday morning to Sunday night he could be called to the hospital anytime to evaluate and possibly operate on patients with serious illnesses.

On Saturday evening when Dr. Smith was on call, Jim Lavalier, 65, was sent to the hospital by his family doctor, Dr. Rosen, because he had stomach pains, bloating, and vomiting—all possible signs of a partially blocked colon (large intestine). Jim was admitted to the hospital by the surgical resident on duty, a surgeon-in-training with 3 years' experience after medical school. The resident phoned Dr. Smith to report that Jim's conditions did not seem to be an emergency. Dr. Smith requested that Jim receive intravenous fluids and pain medication during the night and planned to see him Sunday morning.

41

Despite performing two late-night operations on Saturday, Dr. Smith went to see Jim late Sunday morning and reviewed his test results. Jim told Dr. Smith that his overall health had been gradually worsening for several months. He had felt weak and been having belly pains nearly every week. His appetite decreased and he had lost about 10 pounds over the past 2 months. To assess his risk for heart problems during surgery, Dr. Smith asked Jim if he had had any previous heart condition. Jim replied that his heart had always been fine. As an after-thought, Jim later mentioned that he had experienced an irregular heartbeat once several years ago that had gone away on its own. He admitted to smoking two packs of cigarettes a day and not exercising much.

At Dr. Smith's request, Jim underwent an examination of his colon via a flex-ible lighted tube introduced through his anus (colonoscopy) on Sunday after-noon. This test revealed that the lower end of the colon was nearly blocked by tissue. Several small samples of the tissue were removed and quickly analyzed using a frozen section technique. Dr. Smith was informed that the colon cells were abnormal, but because of the very small size of the biopsies, it was not pos-sible to clearly establish if that abnormality was cancerous. Thus Dr. Smith could not be certain at this point if the blockage was due to a growing cancer or diverticulitis—a severe inflammation of the colon.

Dr. Smith knew that a computed tomographic (CT) scan of the abdomen could help clarify Jim's condition and provide information about the location of other vital organs in the area. Obtaining the CT scan had two important drawbacks, however. The scan would cost $600 ($200 more expensive on week-ends) and Jim's insurance carrier, a regional Health Maintenance Organization (HMO), probably would disallow the charge for the scan as they often did for expensive x-ray tests. Dr. Smith also knew that if he ordered CT scans for what the insurance carrier considered to be too many of his patients, the HMO could cancel its contract with his practice group and the flow of patients and associ-ated income into his practice and the hospital would decrease. After considering these factors, Dr. Smith decided that although the CT scan might be helpful, he would not order it and instead would rely on his experience in colon surgery to avoid complications.

Dr. Smith knew that Jim's partial colon blockage required surgery and al-though it was not an emergency—it could safely wait 24 hours—he decided that adding this operation to the already-full Monday schedule would be too disrup-tive to patients and the operating room (OR) staff because of the possibility of having to delay or cancel already scheduled operations to accommodate Jim's surgery. He would proceed with Jim's surgery on Sunday night despite being tired from performing two operations the night before and having slept a total of only 4 hours since Saturday. Dr. Smith talked with Jim, describing the sur-gery and the possibility of complications including infection, damage to other organs, and bleeding. Dr. Smith told Jim that one of the risks of this operation is cutting the ureter—a small muscular tube that brings the urine from the kidney to the bladder. Jim seemed to understand and signed the informed consent form required by law in every state. After talking to Jim, Dr. Smith sipped a cup of strong coffee and to overcome his fatigue and slight irritability, focused on Jim's operation. He had missed dinner while evaluating Jim's condition; to appease his hunger, he grabbed a few crackers from the nurses' lounge just before entering the OR.

The mood in the OR was somewhat sour because of the large number of weekend surgeries that had taken place and scheduling Jim's surgery for the late hour on Sunday. Dr. Susan Holmes, the anesthesiologist, could not find Jim's old medical chart so she asked him routine questions about his medical condition to determine his risk for anesthesia. Jim, nervous about his surgery, failed to mention his irregular heartbeat problem to Dr. Holmes. It happened that Dr. Smith was scrubbing his hands at that moment and also forgot to mention the irregular heartbeat to Dr. Holmes. He assumed Dr. Holmes would obtain all the necessary the information about Jim and take the necessary precautions to avoid problems during surgery. The physical conditions in the OR were also mildly unpleasant as usual—the room was kept cold to reduce the sweating caused by the impermeable gowns worn by the surgeons—which added to Dr. Smith's annoyance.

After Jim was under anesthesia and the surgical site sterilized and draped, Dr. Smith took the scalpel and made the incision in the abdominal wall. This is open surgery as illustrated in Fig. 4.1; Jim Lavalier's problem was not amenable to a minimally invasive, laparoscopic procedure. As he was proceeding, Dr. Smith remembered to ask if Jim had received the antibiotics to prevent infection in the wound that he had ordered to be given just before surgery. Dr. Holmes informed Dr. Smith that it was not her duty to administer antibiotics; the nurses on the ward should have administered them before surgery. She checked Jim's chart to determine if that had been done and found the vial of antibiotics taped to the front cover, apparently with the presumption that the medication would given in the OR. Dr. Smith was annoyed that this important and scientifically established measure to prevent infection after surgery was missed due to poor communication and asked that the antibiotics be administered immediately even though the optimum time for their administration had passed.

The Sunday evening staffing in the operating room is always less reliable than during the workweek; the circulating nurse that evening was inexperienced and a bit overwhelmed by the many tasks needed to get Jim properly prepared for anesthesia after his arrival in the OR. One of the tasks was placing a 4 × 6-inch adhesive grounding pad on Jim's right thigh to safely conduct the electricity from the electrocautery machine (a device that uses electricity to cut tissue and coagulate small blood vessels at the same time) away from his body.

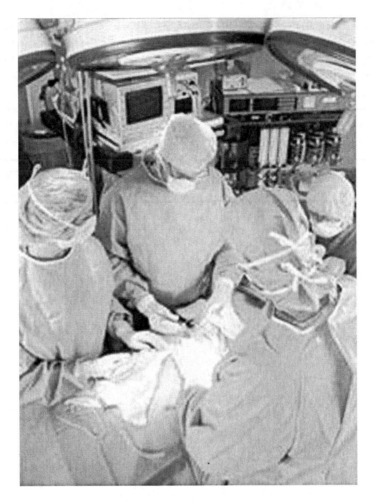

FIG. 4.1.   Open surgery.

Dr. Smith was anxious to get started and to save time, so he hurriedly placed the pad on Jim's thigh instead of waiting for the circulating nurse to do it.

Dr. Smith began the operation and as he squinted into the depths of Jim's abdominal cavity, he noticed dimness in the overhead surgical light. The nurse informed him that one of the two OR lights had a broken bulb that would not be replaced until Monday, and he would need to wear a fiber optic light on a headband to better illuminate the surgical site. The headlight band felt tight around his forehead and the fiber optic cable extending down his back occasionally pulled on his neck. Already tired, the accumulation of physical annoyances caused his back and neck to ache not long after surgery commenced.

As he routinely cut and dissected Jim's internal tissues, Dr. Smith was making decisions about his overall action plan. He still was not sure whether Jim's blockage was caused by a cancer in the bowel or inflammation in the bowel from diverticulitis. If it was cancer, then he must remove more bowel and tissue to assure a cure. To play it safe, he decided to perform the more extensive cancer surgery, knowing that one of the critical steps during this more extended operation is to separate the colon from the ureter, which lies just behind the colon itself, without injuring it. During this time, there was a substantial amount of noise from various alarms on the anesthesia machine, from the suction tubing Dr. Smith was using to aspirate blood and fluid from the surgical field, from the patient air warmer, and the ever-present chatter of the circulating nurses.

Tired and anxious to complete the operation as well as a bit distracted by the noise, Dr. Smith cut through the thickened tissue around the area of the blockage and at one point noticed clear yellow fluid flowing out a small tubular structure. Instantly, Dr. Smith realized that he had inadvertently done exactly what he was trying to avoid: He cut the ureter. To repair this unintended injury, Dr. James, the urologist, was called at home to come to the hospital to perform the delicate repair. Dr. James' repair was successful but it added 2 hours to the duration of Jim's surgery. During this additional time, Jim's heart began to exhibit some extra beats and Dr. Holmes had to administer a heart medication to regulate the beats. After things stabilized, Dr. Smith completed the removal of the colon without further incident.

When the surgical drapes were removed from Jim's body, the circulating nurse in the OR called Dr. Smith's attention to a reddish area on Jim's thigh where the grounding pad for the electrocautery machine had been placed. The pad had partially separated from the skin possibly due to incorrect application before surgery. Dr. Smith recognized the signs of a second-degree burn in the area and knew that this incident would require a formal report the next day and the injury, though not severe, would be painful and take several weeks to heal with a visible scar.

Jim initially recovered well, but 3 days after surgery he developed abdominal pain, fever, and a rapid heart rate and was found to have an infection in the surgical incision. This required removing the skin stitches and leaving the tissues down to the muscle open to drain and heal on their own over several months. Jim's recovery continued to be difficult, requiring a 5-day stay in the intensive care unit because of a mild heart attack, triggered by a rapid and irregular heartbeat possibly related to the stress of the infection. Ultimately, after 12 days, Jim was discharged from the hospital with a contract for home nursing services to provide dressing care for his open wound and to assist him with the physical recovery from his hospital stay.

The complications during Jim's treatment—a cut ureter, a wound infection, and a heart attack—required peer-review according to hospital and regulatory policy. Dr. Smith presented Jim's case for comment to a group of nurses and physicians during the monthly Morbidity and Mortality conference (M&M; morbidity refers to nonfatal complications or adverse events). Some of his colleagues suggested that a CT scan of the abdomen before surgery might have alerted Dr. Smith to the dense scar tissue around the ureter and suggested other safety measures to avoid injuring this structure.

The chief of anesthesiology commented on the fact that Dr. Holmes did not elicit the history of rapid heartbeat from Jim and that Dr. Smith failed to tell her about it. All participants agreed that the preventative antibiotics should have been given before surgery, but no one was sure exactly who was responsible for doing this. Despite the mishaps during Jim's treatment, the participants felt that Dr. Smith had generally practiced within the standard of care—the expected level of care from reasonable physicians in the surrounding community—and had not shown any gross negligence. The report from this conference was protected from public discovery by law and filed with the hospital administration. Nevertheless, Dr. Smith felt responsible for the decisions, technical complications, and the communication failures that had ultimately played an important role in Jim's difficult recovery.

Jim recovered from his illness, but it had been a harrowing experience that left him changed forever. The cost of his care amounted to $75,000. Dr. Smith knew that his fatigue and the timing of the surgery had affected his judgment. He felt he should have remembered to ask for the antibiotics before he made the incision, and if he had told Dr. Holmes about Jim's history of an irregular heartbeat, preventative medications might have been given that would have avoided his heart attack. He felt he had tried his best under physically and mentally demanding conditions, and yet the patient suffered serious complications. Dr. Smith wondered if he could continue to practice with confidence after this ordeal. He sought out the opinion of Dr. Adams, one of his more senior colleagues. Dr. Adams listened calmly to Dr. Smith's difficulties with Jim's case and said in an understanding tone and a slightly world-weary voice: "Welcome to the club, Bob."

MEDICAL ERRORS IN SURGERY: BACKGROUND

Surgery and surgical care are expensive and involve complex interactions among providers, patients, and other health care components. Complications such as bleeding, infection, and technical problems have long been considered an unavoidable part of surgery—and acceptable if kept to a minimum by vigilance and proper training on the part of the surgeon (Greenfield, 1990).

The patient safety movement has gained momentum with the establishment of the National Patient Safety Foundation (Goldsmith, 1997; Kern, 1998). The analysis of iatrogenic complications (adverse outcomes suffered by patients related to the treatment they received) has shifted focus from a provider-centered approach (blaming the person responsible for the care) to a systems-based approach of understanding human error as a consequence of the interaction of the person with the environment (Bogner, 1994). A 1999 report from the Institute of Medicine (IOM) estimated that 2% to 4% of all patients admitted to hospitals in the United States experienced an adverse outcome associated with an adverse event (Kohn, Corrigan, & Donaldson, 2000). Of those events, about half were considered to be preventable and one quarter of those were judged to be possibly negligent. Chillingly, the IOM report estimated that 40,000 to 90,000 patient deaths occur each year due to adverse events presumably caused by human error in the delivery of health care.

Very little information is available on medical error and adverse events in the field of surgery. In 1981, 1% of 5,612 surgical admissions suffered a serious adverse event with a resulting 50% mortality and an average excess hospitalization of 40 days (Couch, Tilney, Rayner, & Moore, 1981). Sixty-two percent of those adverse events involved errors of commission, with the remainder being errors of omission. In 1997, 46% of 1,047 surgical patients experienced an adverse event, one quarter of which were life or limb threatening (Andrews et al., 1997). Individuals were identified as being responsible for less than 38% of the errors, with the remainder being intrinsic to the provision of health care. Most recently, the IOM report stated that 48% (Brennan et al., 1991; Leape et al., 1991) and 35% (Thomas et al., 1999) of all adverse events were associated with surgical care. Infection, bleeding, and technical complications were the most common types of surgical complications.

This chapter explores salient issues relevant to adverse patient events in surgical care (surgical complications) by discussing the interconnected components involved in delivering health care that affect patient safety and the effective delivery of quality care.

Patient Factors

Surgeons know that poor wound healing and infection are common complications following surgery. Patient factors such as poor appetite, weight loss, smoking, drug abuse, and anemia (low blood count) are important conditions that impair the body's ability to heal and that leave the patient susceptible to infection (Sabiston & Lyerly, 1997). This means that even the correct diagnosis and a flawless operation can result in serious complications to the patient if tissues do not heal and the ever-present bacteria in our environment overwhelm the body's natural defenses. Although surgeons have some tools at their disposal such as blood transfusion and intravenous nutrition to help fortify a weakened patient, these avenues are not always appropriate or timely. Ultimately, it is the patient's own body that has to heal and recover from surgery. In Jim's case, his poor nutrition from lack of eating, his previous irregular heartbeat, as well as his smoking habit and lack of exercise, were established conditions that predisposed him to complications—conditions that were unalterable in the short term and that Drs. Smith and Holmes had to accept as part of the risk of treatment.

Cost-of-Care Considerations

Changes in U.S. health care from practitioner-driven to managed care have occurred due to the need to limit the costs of medical care (Kraus, Porter, & Ball, 1990). Thus, cost considerations impact the decision-making process in medicine and surgery (Varney & Schroeder, 1990). Requests for expensive tests that might provide additional information are carefully scrutinized by third-party payers to determine if they are absolutely necessary. Sometimes alternative and lower cost tests are suggested (such as an ultrasound test instead of a CT scan) or the tests are disallowed altogether. In the latter situation, the burden of the cost of tests for the patient rests on the patient, or on the hospital if the patient is unable to pay. The consequence of this process is that hospitals and third-party payers review practice profiles of individual physicians and penalize those who spend more money on tests than the average. This penalty may result in warnings or discontinuation of association between a payer and a physician, with the resultant loss of work and income from being denied access to care for that payer's insured patient population. Dr. Smith decided not to get a CT scan on Jim before surgery primarily because of this, in addition to anticipated delays in availability of the test on weekends and his training that makes him feel a CT scan was not absolutely necessary. Certainly, most diagnostic decisions are not made on the basis of cost alone, yet this factor can be important in medical decision making when added to other factors discussed in this chapter.

Information

Surgical diagnosis is an inexact science. The surgeon is faced with having to make a definitive decision about the need for surgery and the type of operation to perform without having complete information at hand on the patient's condition (Steele, Eiseman, & Norton, 1993). This incomplete dataset may be due to one or more of the following factors: no diagnostic test is available, available tests have a measurable inaccuracy (the level of detail that an x-ray test can deliver is limited to abnormalities that are about one centimeter in size), logistical obstacles to scheduling and performing some complex tests, the cost of the tests, the physical risk to the patient of the test, the patient being uncooperative or giving a poor medical history, and incomplete, illegible, or unavailable patient's records.

In Dr. Smith's case, Jim gave incomplete information on his previous heart condition, and Dr. Holmes did not have the medical record to review prior to anesthesia. Cost and efficiency considerations led Dr. Smith to not perform a CT scan on Jim before surgery, limiting the information he had at hand to plan the surgical procedure. The need to obtain a quick result on the biopsy with a frozen section limited the diagnostic ability of the pathologist to tell whether Jim had cancer. This in turn affected Dr. Smith's decision to perform a more extensive cancer surgery in case the problem was cancer, which increased the probability of injuring the ureter during dissection.

Diagnostic Dilemmas.   During the recovery period following surgery, the surgeon is faced again with diagnostic dilemmas and incomplete information. A sudden drop in the patient's blood pressure may be due to a heart attack, a blood clot in the lungs, or internal bleeding. A heart attack or a blood clot each requires a different type of medical treatment; internal bleeding necessitates a rapid return to surgery. Simple bedside tests such as electrocardiograms, x-rays of the chest, and blood counts can begin to clarify the situation, yet the picture is not always clear. In Jim's case, Dr. Smith had to decide whether the fever, abdominal pain, and elevated heart rate were due to an infection in several possible locations including the lungs, the bladder, inside the abdomen, or in the surgical wound.

The consequences of reaching the wrong conclusion can be serious. For example, using a blood thinner for a suspected blood clot in a patient who is actually bleeding can be fatal. Similarly, emergency surgery for presumed bleeding in a patient actually suffering from a blood clot can have serious adverse consequences. To attain a higher degree of diagnostic certainty, further testing may be needed involving higher risks, higher costs, and more time. The surgeon must continually balance the quality of information available at each moment with the risk and benefit to the patient of either acquiring more information or proceeding directly with treatment. While many, if not most, medical situations can be interpreted correctly and treated promptly with modern diagnostic means, the proper care of a surgical patient is always a less-than-exact process that is influenced by many different health care factors.

Dealing With Adverse Events

When Dr. Adams, Dr. Smith's senior colleague, said, "Welcome to the club," he was referring to the reality that complications are an unavoidable part of surgical practice. Every experienced surgeon knows that between the error-provoking conditions in the process of performing surgery and the many inefficiencies and glitches in health care (unreadable handwriting in physicians' orders, delays in nursing care due to understaffing and sudden emergencies, delays in transcription of test results), things are going to go wrong with a certain regularity. Practicing surgeons know that try as they may to avoid them, adverse events will occur. The time-honored system used to supervise the quality of care in medicine is the use of regular institutional M&M conferences (Gordon, 1994). The purpose of this conference is to review complications that have occurred during a recent period of time and to discuss what could be done to avoid them in the future.

M&M Conferences.   The participants in the M&M conference include surgeons and related hospital staff such as the OR supervisor and the chief of anesthesia (other medical and surgical specialties have their own M&M conferences). Surgeons tend to be very understanding of the myriad of problems that arise outside the control of their peers; however, they are most critical of perceived errors in judgment and decision making. Purely technical mistakes are felt to be uncommon. Discussions at M&M conferences typically focus on the thought process of diagnosis and treatment of surgical patients. Deviations from the local standard of care are discussed and recommendations for improvement are made. Complications are graded by the presiding department chief as unpreventable, possibly preventable, or preventable. Other coding systems may be used that assign levels of conformity to or deviation from the local standard of care. The end result can be a negative review of the case under discussion that is placed in the surgeon's file, along with the embarrassment of exposure of a misjudgment to his or her peers.

Depending on the participants, an M&M conference may be very benign or very malignant. Leading academic institutions have long had a history of malignant M&M conferences where surgical trainees and junior staff members are raked over the coals by senior staff for the complications in their cases. These hazings often are biased by the beliefs of the dominant department members for the point under discussion, rather than being based solely on scientific evidence. The opposite may happen in small community hospitals where independently practicing surgeons are reluctant to criticize their peers in an open setting. In these circumstances, significant errors in judgment or technique can be overlooked or tolerated for social or political reasons. Dr. Smith's experience was somewhere between these two extremes. He was criticized for not obtaining a preoperative CT scan; however, his peers recognized that he had little control over who administered antibiotics once they were ordered appropriately. Dr. Smith was aware of the many competing pressures that led him to make each decision in Jim's case. Although he believed that no one decision had been wrong, lazy, or overtly dangerous, he realized that each small compromise had ultimately played a role in the outcome of Jim's care.

MENTAL AND PHYSICAL STRESS
IN SURGICAL PRACTICE

Surgeons train in residency programs based on a mentorship system for a period of 5 to 6 years. Residency training consists of an intensive exposure to diseases that require surgery for treatment and provides technical training in performing these operations and caring for the patients before and after surgery ("National surgical work patterns as a basis for residency training plans: the response of a panel of surgeons," 1977). Residents' work schedules are frequently 80 to 120 hours per week and are justified by the argument that this exposure maximizes the intensity of the learning and accustoms the residents to overcoming fatigue when dealing with serious illness. In other words, residents are trained to always place the necessities of patients' care above their own comfort and needs (Bunch, Dvonch, Storr, Baldwin, & Hughes, 1992).

Although this highly driven and chronically sleep-deprived work schedule has been suspected to lead to errors in judgment, planning, and execution of surgical procedures by residents, it remains unclear just how much performance impairment from sleep deprivation and frequent on-call schedules occurs. Certainly, this work regimen results in alterations in mood such as anger and frustration among overworked residents (Bartle et al., 1988; Brown, 1994; Sawyer, Tribble, Newberg, Pruett, & Minasi, 1999).

In Dr. Smith's case, members of his practice group routinely take a 3-day weekend call even with the possibility of having to perform surgery each night. Not only does Dr. Smith's schedule risk fatigue during the weekend, but he also is likely to begin the next work week in less than optimal physical and mental condition to perform critical decisions and procedures. In the case of Jim's surgery, Dr. Smith performed two operations the night before that had left him tired and likely less adaptable and open in his decision-making skills. Although Dr. Smith attempted to sharpen his cognitive processes by drinking coffee, his fatigue, lack of proper food, and the frustrations of communication and ambient distractions in the OR simply ganged up on him. The reader can sense how Dr. Smith's decision making, interpersonal skills and manual skills were all subtly affected by the stress of his working conditions.

Error

Medicine approaches human error from the traditional point of view of individual responsibility and has established a culture of blame surrounding adverse events. In surgical training, it is the norm that the surgeons should assume all the responsibility for the patient's care. They are trained to feel completely responsible for everything that does and does not happen to their patients. This extreme view of responsibility drives dedicated surgeons to attempt to mitigate the risks of health care by working to correct or prevent errors and absorbing their effects when they happen.

No matter what the events leading up to an operation were, and no matter how error-provoking the conditions at the time of surgery might be, the surgeon is expected to carry out the operation successfully and pull the patient through. Often this means absorbing a large amount of physical and mental stress. It also means that the operation often is not performed under optimal, or even desirable, mental and physical circumstances. Behind the surgeon's strong sense of commitment to the patient, instilled by years of training, is the ever-present specter of malpractice litigation. Although this view of individual responsibility makes the physician a strong personal advocate for the care of each patient, the elevated expectation of individual responsibility and performance in the midst of recognizably unsafe conditions of medical care can be very frustrating.

THE OR ENVIRONMENT

Surgery had its origins on kitchen tables and in courtyards and gradually evolved to having a workspace of its own: the OR (Bishop, 1960). The first operating rooms were simply large, well-lit rooms or amphitheaters where surgery could be performed with just a few instruments. Surgery has always been messy work, associated with pain, infection, body fluids, and the struggle to accomplish the goal. The advent of anesthesia and the concepts of asepsis at the end of the 19th century launched the modern era of surgery (Billings, 1970). Over the past 100 years, operations have come from being a dreaded treatment of last resort to routinely planned interventions with great attention to minimizing pain and suffering. Despite this evolution, the OR remains a potentially dangerous workplace for the OR team with risks posed by infection (Jagger & Perry, 2000), electrical current (Litt & Ehrenwerth, 1994), and large equipment items such as portable X-ray machines (Laufman, 1976), as well as physical discomforts due to the cold temperature (Weinger & Englund, 1990), high noise levels from equipment (Hodge & Thompson, 1990), and alarms (Loeb, Jones, Leonard, & Behrman, 1992). Decreasing the environmental hazards in the OR is a recognized goal (Laufman, 1994).

The danger of doing harm is lurking behind every move the surgeon makes. A torn blood vessel, a severed nerve, or a spill of infected body fluids into an otherwise sterile area can occur at any moment and with the slightest distraction.

This is not to say that surgery demands undivided concentration at all times, but rather that the consequences of distraction or disorientation at critical points in the operation can have severe consequences for the patient and for the surgeon. It is important to recognize, then, that surgeons are exposed to significant environmental distractions and even hazards, not the least of which are awkward body postures trying to view and manipulate internal body parts (Kant, de Jong, van Rijssen-Moll, & Borm, 1992). Dr. Smith struggled with many of these factors in addition to poor lighting. The result of these environmental factors diminishes the mental and physical reserve that the surgeon needs to make appropriate decisions and to carry out technically correct maneuvers.

Communication and Teamwork

The work of health care providers involved in surgery necessitates their working as a team—a group of individuals with a common goal. Teams work best when appropriate training in procedures and communication are given (Klein, 1986). In the OR, surgical teams consist of members of three professions—nursing, anesthesiology, and surgery—who typically are not trained specifically to work as a team (Helmreich & Musson, 2000). Members of each of those professions acquire their professional skills through separate graduate training programs, only interacting in the context of actually performing surgery (whether during training or clinical practice). It is no surprise, therefore, that communication between anesthesiologists and surgeons before an operation often is deficient. This can result in unexpected delays because key information about the patient's medical condition or the specific plans for surgery is missing. Dr. Smith forgot to pass on the information about Jim's previous heart condition to Dr. Holmes, an omission that was aided by the lack of availability of Jim's medical records and the fallibility of taking his medical history orally. Dr. Smith did not discuss his specific surgical plans with Dr. Holmes, including the potential risks of cutting a ureter with the attendant possibility of an additional 2 hours of anesthetic time to repair it. Conveying this information may not have seemed relevant to Dr. Smith, but it might have helped Dr. Holmes better plan the anesthetic management and prepare for unexpected events such as Jim's rapid heartbeat during surgery.

The relevance of team research in other medical and nonmedical domains to the OR is clear. A comparison of attitudes toward teamwork in operating rooms, intensive care units, and major airlines concluded that physicians and nurses find error comparatively more difficult to discuss in medical settings, and medical staff often deny the effect of stress and fatigue on their performance (Sexton, Thomas, & Helmreich, 2000). Other problems experienced by OR personnel are differing perceptions of teamwork among team members and reluctance of senior operating theatre staff to accept input from junior members. In emergency medicine, a team approach with proper training can decrease errors and the cost of emergency medical care (Risser et al., 1999; Small et al., 1999). A trained nursing team facilitates laparoscopic surgical procedures—surgery performed through a "keyhole" incision using a telescope and a video camera to project images of the inside of the body on a TV screen (Kenyon, Lenker, Bax, & Swanstrom, 1997).

Scheduling

Surgeons do not work in a vacuum. The process of diagnosing and treating patients with surgical disease requires the coordination of people and tests from different medical departments. Often the process is linear in nature such that the results of one test dictate the need for another. Modern hospitals are busy places and the efficient scheduling of tests and surgical procedures can be a challenging task (Blake & Carter, 1997). In Dr. Smith's case, his choice of operating on Sunday night under less-than-ideal circumstances, such as no backup and a tired crew, was dictated partly by Jim's condition and partly by the schedule for the operating room that already was booked for the week. The impact of attempting to perform Jim's surgery on Monday morning would have been a total disruption in the work of dozens of people. This decision, however, imposed time pressures such as making a CT scan less practical because the delay for a technician on Sunday is greater than during the week.

An alternative safety strategy for preventing damage to the ureter would have been to ask Dr. James to come to the hospital to place ureteral stents (small plastic tubes) in Jim just before the start of surgery to help Dr. Smith identify—and not injure—the structure during the difficult dissection. The late-night surgery on Sunday made this undesirable. It is often the case that the combined pressures of scheduling and cost containment lead to treatment decisions that are compromised compared to optimum standards (Steele et al., 1993).

Balancing Diverse Needs.   Management of the OR strives to balance the needs of patients, the staff, the hospital, and the external regulatory agencies (Barratt & Schultz, 1997). There are no standardized routines for OR scheduling (Blake & Carter, 1997), and each institution strives to maximize the utilization of its resources while providing a safe and effective environment for surgery. For example, surgeons are required to book their cases ahead of time and provide a reasonable time estimate for the length of the operations. This time estimate is highly variable because some surgeons work faster than others, and many are not good judges of their own speed. Adding to the complexity is the fact that unexpected findings or intraoperative complications (complications during surgery) are not uncommon and may require substantial additional surgical time. The addition of urgent and emergency operations to the day or evening schedule further disrupts the scheduling process and taxes the OR human resources.

Dr. Smith could have decided to perform Jim's operation the following day when he was more rested, when Jim's medical records were likely to have been found, and when there were more support staff for unexpected occurrences during surgery. Yet Dr. Smith knew that the addition of a single urgent operation into that day's already full OR schedule would delay every operation. This would mean that the last scheduled cases of the day might be delayed to the extent that OR staff would be required to work extended shifts to finish the day's work. Alternatively, other operations might have to be cancelled and rescheduled, creating frustration among the patients and their doctors. Dr. Smith was aware of these factors, which influenced his decision that it would be most efficient for the OR as a whole to proceed with Jim's operation on Sunday night despite being tired and the lack of available help for unexpected problems.

Technology in the OR

Surgery has become increasingly technology-dependent (Mathias, 1992). Even a simple task such as cutting tissue is routinely performed with instruments such as electrocautery, ultrasonic "scalpels," and lasers. These devices help reduce blood loss by coagulating bleeding vessels and generally make the operation proceed faster. At the same time, they introduce new risks to the patient and the OR staff. Electrocautery machines use high-voltage electrical currents passing through a hand-held probe to the patient's tissues to cut tissue while closing off small bleeding vessels. These devices (also called Bovies) require proper grounding of the patient to allow the current to flow through his or her body without injury.

When the grounding is faulty, a burn can occur where electricity exits the body toward a natural ground (Wald, Mazzia, & Spencer, 1971; Zinder & Parker, 1996). Dr. Smith placed the electrocautery grounding pad himself because he was in a rush, but he had not been trained to do this simple procedure. He thought it simply had to be placed on the thigh; he did not realize that certain locations are preferable because they lessen the chance that the pad will come off during surgery and result in a burn. When Jim was awakened and the drapes removed, the nurse noted the pad had partially separated from Jim's skin and that a burn had occurred at this location. There are a number of possible causes of this problem including incorrect location or application of the pad, partial removal of the pad due to movement of the patient during induction of anesthesia, sweating and loosening of the pad adhesive, etc. In Dr. Smith's case, impatience, poor team communication, and lack of training in a simple procedure resulted in an unexpected injury to the patient.

CONCLUSION

Surgeons, more than medical physicians, work in a complex, demanding, and potentially hazardous environment. The nature of surgery (and other invasive procedures such as heart catheterization) requires the surgeon to cause a calculated amount of harm to the patient (pain, scarring, inflammation) in order to bring about a greater good such as removing a cancer or repairing a painful hernia. This decision to directly invade a patient's body has a subtle but profound impact on surgeons' relationship with their patients and their sense of responsibility.

As they interact with the OR and other aspects of the hospital, surgeons must balance scheduling efficiency and cost containment while at the same time feeling completely responsible for the care of their patients. Decision making is central to good surgical care, yet it often must be carried out with insufficient and inexact information. Surgeons generally place their own safety and comfort second to patients' welfare and often are overworked and sleep deprived due to the demands of on-call surgery. The surgeons' home territory—the OR—far from being a safe haven, can be a noisy, uncomfortable, and sometimes hazardous place to work. The lack of team training and communication skills can create delays, miscommunication, and interpersonal friction among surgeons, nurses, and anesthesiologists.

This chapter afforded the reader a glimpse into the surgeon's world with its many error-provoking factors—a world unknown to the layperson. As medicine in the United States changes, with more and more surgeons working as salaried employees whose performance will be scrutinized by administrators, the tradition of the stoic and independent surgeon is gradually changing. These and other developments portend a new era where surgeons will recognize the effects of fatigue on performance, accept outside monitoring of the quality of their surgical care, and readily participate in open and multidisciplinary efforts to rid the health care system of its many sources of system errors. Significant improvements in the safety of health care for patients as well as providers will not occur until the factors that negatively affect surgeons' performance are understood and rectified.

REFERENCES

Andrews, L. B., Stocking, C., Krizek, T., Gottlieb, L., Krizek, C., Vargish, T., & Siegler, M. (1997). An alternative strategy for studying adverse events in medical care [see comments]. *Lancet, 349*(9048), 309–313.

Barratt, C. C., & Schultz, M. K. (1997). Staffing the operating room. Time and space factors. *Journal of Nursing Administration, 27*(12), 27–31.

Bartle, E. J., Sun, J. H., Thompson, L., Light, A. I., McCool, C., & Heaton, S. (1988). The effects of acute sleep deprivation during residency training. *Surgery, 104*(2), 311–316.

Billings, J. S. (1970). *The history and literature of surgery.* New York: Argosy-Antiquarian.

Bishop, W. J. (1960). *The early history of surgery.* London: R. Hale.

Blake, J. T., & Carter, M. W. (1997). Surgical process scheduling: A structured review. *Journal of the Society for Health Systems, 5*(3), 17–30.

Bogner, M. S. (1994). *Human error in medicine.* Hillsdale, NJ: Lawrence Erlbaum Associates.

Brennan, T. A., Leape, L. L., Laird, N. M., Hebert, L., Localio, A. R., Lawthers, A. G., Newhouse, J. P., Weiler, P. C., & Hiatt, H. H. (1991). Incidence of adverse events and negligence in hospitalized patients. Results of the Harvard Medical Practice Study I. *New England Journal of Medicine, 324*(6), 370–376.

Brown, I. D. (1994). Driver fatigue. *Human Factors, 36*(2), 298–314.

Bunch, W. H., Dvonch, V. M., Storr, C. L., Baldwin, D. C. Jr., & Hughes, P. H. (1992). The stresses of the surgical residency. *Journal of Surgical Research, 53*(3), 268–271.

Couch, N. P., Tilney, N. L., Rayner, A. A., & Moore, F. D. (1981). The high cost of low-frequency events: The anatomy and economics of surgical mishaps. *New England Journal of Medicine, 304*(11), 634–637.

Goldsmith, M. F. (1997). National Patient Safety Foundation studies systems [news]. *Journal of the American Medical Association, 278*(19), 1561.

Gordon, L. A. (1994). *Gordon's guide to the surgical morbidity and mortality conference.* Philadelphia: Hanley & Belfus.

Greenfield, L. J. (1990). *Complications in surgery and trauma* (2nd ed.). Philadelphia: Lippincott.

Helmreich, R. L., & Musson, D. M. (2000). Surgery as team endeavour [editorial]. *Canadian Journal of Anaesthesia, 47*(5), 391–392.

Hodge, B., & Thompson, J. F. (1990). Noise pollution in the operating theatre. *Lancet, 335,* 891–894.

Jagger, J., & Perry, J. (2000). Safety in the OR. *Nursing, 30*(8), 77.

Kant, I. J., de Jong, L. C., van Rijssen-Moll, M., & Borm, P. J. (1992). A survey of static and dynamic work postures of operating room staff. *International Archives of Occupational and Environmental Health, 63*(6), 423–428.

Kenyon, T. A., Lenker, M. P., Bax, T. W., & Swanstrom, L. L. (1997). Cost and benefit of the trained laparoscopic team. A comparative study of a designated nursing team vs a nontrained team. *Surgical Endoscopy, 11*(8), 812–814.

Kern, K. A. (1998). The National Patient Safety Foundation: What it offers surgeons. *Bulletin of the American College of Surgeons, 83*(11), 24–27, 46.

Klein, G. (1986). The art of leadership in management. *Trends and Techniques in the Contemporary Dental Laboratory, 3*(3), 2, 4–6, 8–10.

Kohn, L. T., Corrigan, J., & Donaldson, M. S. (2000). *To err is human: Building a safer health system.* Washington, DC: National Academy Press.

Kraus, N., Porter, M., & Ball, P. (1990). *Managed care: A decade in review, 1980–1990* (Special ed.). Excelsior, MN: InterStudy.

Laufman, H. (1976). Trends in operating room devices. *Medical Instrumentation, 10*(2), 98–104.

Laufman, H. (1994). Streamlining environmental safety in the operating room: A common bond between surgeons and hospital engineers. *Healthcare Facilities Management and Service,* 1–14.

Leape, L. L., Brennan, T. A., Laird, N., Lawthers, A. G., Localio, A. R., Barnes, B. A., Hebert, L., Newhouse, J. P., Weiler, P. C., & Hiatt, H. (1991). The nature of adverse events in hospitalized patients. Results of the Harvard Medical Practice Study II. *New England Journal of Medicine, 324*(6), 377–384.

Litt, L., & Ehrenwerth, J. (1994). Electrical safety in the operating room: Important old wine, disguised new bottles [editorial; comment]. *Anesthesia and Analgesia, 78*(3), 417–419.

Loeb, R. G., Jones, B. R., Leonard, R. A., & Behrman, K. (1992). Recognition accuracy of current operating room alarms. *Anesthesia and Analgesia, 75*(4), 499–505.

Mathias, J. M. (1992). Advanced technology in the operating room. *OR Manager, 8*(5), 10–13.

National surgical work patterns as a basis for residency training plans: the response of a panel of surgeons. (1977). *Archives of Surgery, 112*(2), 125–147.

Risser, D. T., Rice, M. M., Salisbury, M. L., Simon, R., Jay, G. D., & Berns, S. D. (1999). The potential for improved teamwork to reduce medical errors in the emergency department. The MedTeams Research Consortium [see comments]. *Annals of Emergency Medicine, 34*(3), 373–383.

Sabiston, D. C., & Lyerly, H. K. (1997). *Textbook of surgery: The biological basis of modern surgical practice* (15th ed.). Philadelphia: W. B. Saunders.

Sawyer, R. G., Tribble, C. G., Newberg, D. S., Pruett, T. L., & Minasi, J. S. (1999). Intern call schedules and their relationship to sleep, operating room participation, stress, and satisfaction. *Surgery, 126*(2), 337–342.

Sexton, J. B., Thomas, E. J., & Helmreich, R. L. (2000). Error, stress, and teamwork in medicine and aviation: cross sectional surveys. *British Medical Journal, 320*(7237), 745–749.

Small, S. D., Wuerz, R. C., Simon, R., Shapiro, N., Conn, A., & Setnik, G. (1999). Demonstration of high-fidelity simulation team training for emergency medicine. *Academic Emergency Medicine, 6*(4), 312–323.

Steele, G., Eiseman, B., & Norton, L. W. (1993). *Surgical decision making* (3rd ed.). Philadelphia: Saunders.

Thomas, E. J., Studdert, D. M., Newhouse, J. P., Zbar, B. I., Howard, K. M., Williams, E. J., & Brennan, T. A. (1999). Costs of medical injuries in Utah and Colorado. *Inquiry, 36*(3), 255–264.

Varney, R. A., & Schroeder, D. J. (1990). "Trade-off" between medical cost controls and quality of care? Maybe, maybe not! Part I. *Journal of Quality Assurance, 12*(1), 10–13, 42.

Wald, A. S., Mazzia, V. D., & Spencer, F. C. (1971). Accidental burns associated with electrocautery. *Journal of the American Medical Association, 217*(7), 916–921.

Weinger, M. B., & Englund, C. E. (1990). Ergonomic and human factors affecting anesthetic vigilance and monitoring performance in the operating room environment [see comments]. *Anesthesiology, 73*(5), 995–1021.

Zinder, D. J., & Parker, G. S. (1996). Electrocautery burns and operator ignorance. *Otolaryngology and Head Neck Surgery, 115*(1), 145–149.

5 Safety and Error Issues in Minimally Invasive Surgery

Christine L. MacKenzie
Alan J. Lomax
Jennifer A. Ibbotson
Simon Fraser University

LAPAROSCOPIC SURGEON, DAVE GARDNER, M.D.

The surgeon, Dave Gardner, was having a hard time. Although he was an experienced and competent surgeon, the minimally invasive (often referred to as keyhole surgery because of the small size of the incisions) laparoscopic cholecystectomy, or gall bladder removal, for Mrs. Sanders was proving to be extremely difficult. The operation started out as usual; Dave made four small incisions, each about half an inch long, in Mrs. Sanders' abdomen. He inserted sharp, pointed instruments called trocars into the incisions and passed a narrow tube several inches long called a cannula through the hole in each trocar into the abdominal cavity. Dave told George Gregory, the resident trainee surgeon who was assisting him, that great care must be used when inserting a trocar because the sharp point on that instrument can injure vital structures in the abdomen. He knew of cases when the large blood vessel called the aorta had been injured when a trocar was inserted, causing the death of the patient; the bowel also can be punctured by a trocar.

As Dave inserted the trocars, he explained to George that he much preferred to use disposable entry instruments because they are always sharp and clean—reusable instruments can have small contaminating particles that remain even after thorough cleaning. Despite his preference, Dave was obliged, on the insistence of the hospital administrator, to perform the procedure with reusable instruments because less cost was involved. Through a trocar, Dave inserted the apparatus that blew carbon dioxide gas into Mrs. Sanders' abdomen; the gas lifted the front of her abdomen creating a space in which the surgical instruments can be used.

Once the cannulae are in place and the abdomen infused with gas, the trocars are removed and the cannulae are used as entrances into Mrs. Sanders' abdominal cavity. The cannulae have valves that keep the carbon dioxide gas from escaping yet allow insertion of the long, thin instruments used in the procedure as well as a tiny telescope attached to a miniature video camera. The camera provides the surgeons an image on a video monitor of the internal structures and the activity of the surgical procedure. Prior to beginning the operation, Dave showed George how the video camera is attached to the telescope and how the cable that brings light to the surgical site inside Mrs. Sanders' abdomen is attached to the camera. Dave switched on the light source and pointed out the bright ring of light that came from the end of the telescope—light that is necessary for the video camera to create the image that is projected on a video monitor.

When Dave started the surgery, he found the gall bladder to be very inflamed. Because of that, the end of the instrument he held in his left hand that was used to grasp tissue would not hold that organ well enough to permit the precise and delicate movements required from the instrument Dave held in his right hand. "Give me the instruments that will do the job," he complained repeatedly. Although those comments apparently were directed to no one in particular, Dave was thinking about the makers of the supposed state-of-the-art instruments he was using.

Dave also was having problems with the clarity of the video monitor picture of the inside of the abdomen and the area where he was operating. For some reason the picture was not as good as it had been during the last laparoscopic gall bladder operation he had performed. He tried refocusing the small video camera on the end of the telescope inside the abdominal cavity. This did not improve the image, so he tried wiping the end of the telescope on Mrs. Sanders' liver. That commonly performed act usually improves the clarity of the picture; however, this time it made no difference. Dave needed a clear image, so as a last resort, he removed the telescope from the cannula in the abdominal wall and asked Debbie Bevens, the operating room nurse, to clean the end. That sterile procedure solved the problem; when the tiny telescope was reinserted through the valve in the cannula, Dave could see the surgical site clearly.

Dave continued with the operation. He withdrew the instrument he held in his right hand from the entry cannula and asked Debbie for a different instrument that he thought would be easier to use. She handed him the instrument; when he tried to insert it, the instrument would not fit in the cannula. Debbie explained that the instrument and cannula were both identified as 5 mm in size but they were made by different companies and obviously were not compatible. Debbie *continued to say that the hospital administration purchased the new instruments from a different company because they cost less. Because of the lack of fit, Dave resumed using the original instrument, inadequate though it was. To add another factor to the situation, the clear video image from cleaning the telescope was only temporary; for Dave to have a clear monitor image of his work, it was necessary for the telescope to be removed repeatedly throughout the operation for Debbie to clean the lens.*

As Dave continued with the difficult surgery, he recalled how he had advised Mrs. Sanders that because of the inflammation in her gall bladder it would be better to perform open surgery. In open surgery, the abdomen is opened with a long incision that would provide better access to the inflamed organ than through the small laparoscopic incisions. Mrs. Sanders insisted that she did not want a large incision through her abdominal wall that would be painful and cause an ugly scar. Also, she had been told by friends that a laparoscopic cholecystectomy is a simple procedure that would enable her to be back at work in a few days. Dave knew that in spite of Mrs. Sanders' refusal to have her gall bladder removed by the safer, open surgery, she would not hesitate to sue him if something went wrong with the laparoscopic procedure.

A sudden shrill beeping sound caught Dave's attention. He asked, "Who stepped on the cautery pedal?" The cautery pedal activates the cautery current, which is electric current passed down surgical instruments that produces heat in the instrument. That heat allows the instrument to be used to control bleeding by sealing the ends of bleeding blood vessels or to cut tissues. Such heat would be dangerous in an unattended instrument, so a beeping sound is produced when the cautery pedal is depressed letting the surgeon know the cautery is active. Debbie replied, "That is not the cautery; it's your pager." So much of the equipment in the operating room has similar warning beeps that it is difficult to identify which beep comes from which piece of equipment. Dave often mistook his pager beep for the very similar cautery warning alarm.

Dave had trouble with another instrument. "These scissors are not cutting— they couldn't cut through butter!" said Dave. "Probably so," said Debbie, "they have been used a lot with cautery." Although the use of the cautery current makes the scissors dull and rather ineffective for cutting, it is very helpful to the surgeon to pass the cautery current down the scissors to control bleeding as well as using the scissors to cut.

As he pressed on the cautery pedal to use it with an instrument, Dave noticed lines of interference on the video monitor and wondered if the electrical insulation at the end of his instrument was defective. He would ask Brian Rogers, the biomedical technician who serviced the instruments, to check it at the end of the operation. Dave was concerned because he knew that there could be unsafe situations when cautery is used. One such situation is when, for no apparent reason, the cautery current could jump from the end of the instrument to other structures in the abdomen that are out of sight of the video camera, such as the bowel, and produce an injury. Such an injury would not be apparent at the time of the operation, although a few days later the injured area of bowel might die and bowel fluid might leak into the abdomen, causing serious complications such as infection.

The very close view of the surgical site that the laparoscopic surgeon has via the lens on the end of the telescope in the abdomen (it is ten times nearer to the operating area than is the surgeon's eye in conventional, open surgery) was helpful for Dave. It magnified the surgical site, which made the structures easier to see; however, the closeness restricted the size of Dave's viewing area. This tunnel vision provided a view of only a small part of the surgical area. With experience, Dave's brain had learned to adapt to the reduced angle of view, which was less than half that of natural vision.

Dave was progressing with the surgery when suddenly the picture on the monitor disappeared. Dave uttered an expletive as he asked what had happened. "I am sorry," said Mary Monroe, the circulating nurse. "I tripped over the camera cable. It must have been loose." The hospital was short-staffed and Mary, who had to work on her scheduled day off, was at the end of her fourth consecutive day of 12-hour shifts. Not only was she tired, Mary was distracted; she was worried about her two young sons who were alone at home with the flu. The camera cable was reattached and the operation continued. Dave often complained about the wires, cables, and tubes connecting the multiple pieces of equipment in the operating room. He also complained about the general clutter in the operating room, which was worse with laparoscopic operations because of the extra equipment necessary for this type of surgery. He believed the obstacles in the operating room constituted an accident waiting to happen.

Because of the inflamed state of the gall bladder, there was more bleeding than usual in the abdominal cavity. Blood not only covered the structures in the operating area but it also absorbed light, making it more difficult for Dave to see what he was doing. In addition, blood stained the various anatomical structures making it difficult to see fine details in the picture on the monitor. Dave inserted the long irrigating tube down one of the cannulae. Out of the end of the tube inside the abdomen came a jet of fluid that cleared away blood that was obscuring the operating area. Dave pressed a button on the irrigating tube and the blood and fluid were then sucked up the tube. It is considerably more difficult to clear the operating area adequately in laparoscopic surgery than it is to clear a surgical site in conventional, open operations. Dave often wished for a better laparoscopic irrigation and suction instrument.

Because of the nature of Mrs. Sanders' problem, the surgery continued to be difficult. The surgery was made more of a challenge by the problems Dave *encountered with the instruments. The instrument in his right hand did not seem to be working well. After struggling with it, he withdrew it from the cannula and saw that the working end was broken. While he was waiting for the nurse to bring a replacement, Dave recalled how difficult he had found laparoscopic procedures when he first began to perform them; it seemed as if his brain was working under great strain. In conventional open surgery, his hands, instruments, and the operating area are all in a straight line and in view. He read that the brain prefers this arrangement, but in minimally invasive surgery, his hands, instruments, and operating area are not in a straight line.*

Laparoscopic surgeons' heads often by necessity are turned away from the instruments to view the picture on the monitor. Their hands, which use handles to manipulate the instruments, receive little if any tactile feedback. In addition, the surgeon's hands most likely are at angles from the internal structures of the operative site, and are a distance from the picture that is, in effect, the operating area—a distance larger than the actual distance of the surgeon's hands from the patient's body. The surgeon's brain finds it more difficult to work with this arrangement than with that of open surgery. In addition, the picture on the monitor is not as clear as the natural vision of conventional open surgery, so it is more difficult to identify small details. Nonetheless, with practice, Dave had quickly learned to perform laparoscopic procedures quite well. A few of his colleagues had not been so fortunate. Although they were excellent surgeons, they could not adapt to that way of operating and with the demand so great for laparoscopic surgery, they had taken early retirement.

Dave found most laparoscopic gall bladder operations easy but not this one. The gall bladder was difficult to hold with the grasper and he could not see clearly because of the bleeding. His laparoscopic instruments would only move in certain directions and he had to assume awkward postures and difficult positions to use them in the way he wished. Normally, he found this not much of a problem but in this difficult case he was beginning to get an aching pain in his wrist and hands. The lack of sensation conveyed to Dave's hands by the end of the laparoscopic instrument about what in the abdominal cavity it is touching, such as the lack of the sensation of pulsation if the instrument is against an artery, makes the procedure more difficult than in open surgery. In open surgery, the instruments are held directly in the surgeon's hands so there is tactile feedback to supplement the surgeon's full view of the surgical site.

Dave was having difficulty in determining the situation of the two vital structures in Mrs. Sanders' surgical area: the cystic duct, a small tube that is attached to the bottom of the gall bladder and passes down to the common bile duct, and the cystic artery situated above the cystic duct. He wished he could put his hand inside the abdomen to feel structures as he did in open surgery. He decided to do a special X-ray known as a cholangiogram to determine the situation with the structures. *This was not successful because of the inflammation and he had to continue without the additional information.*

Dave's main concern was to avoid injury to the common bile duct because he knew this could be devastating. The common bile duct is the tube that carries bile from the liver to the intestines, which is a very important activity. If that were inadvertently cut, Mrs. Sanders would experience problems for the rest of her life. The surgical target Dave was trying to identify is the cystic duct that joins the common bile duct about halfway down; in this case, it was particularly difficult to identify because of the inflammation and swelling.

Eventually Dave identified the cystic duct and artery, placed small metal clips on them, divided them with scissors, removed the gall bladder from under the liver, and withdrew it from the abdomen. The surgery was completed; Dave gave a big sigh of relief. It had been one of the most difficult laparoscopic gall bladder operations he had done. In spite of the difficulties, Dave thought Mrs. Sanders would make an uneventful recovery and return to her job as a receptionist in less than two weeks. Events, however, were to prove him wrong.

Dave was leaving for his vacation the next day and intended to hand over the care of Mrs. Sanders to his colleague Martin Rodgers. Martin was an excellent surgeon and Dave had no concerns about his care of Mrs. Sanders. Dave usually spoke to Martin personally when he left patients in his care, but on this occasion Martin was in the operating room and not available. Rather than wait for him to complete the surgery, Dave wrote a note about Mrs. Sanders and left it for Martin. Unfortunately, a well-meaning person decided to tidy the area and inadvertently threw Dave's note into the trash, so Martin, who had forgotten that Dave was going on vacation, was unaware that Mrs. Sanders was in his care.

In the immediate post-operative period, Mrs. Sanders appeared to make good progress; however, about 24 hours after the operation, she began to have increasing abdominal pain and was given pain medication by the nurse. This seemed to control the pain and the nurse was not unduly concerned. Normally at this stage of recovery, Mrs. Sanders would have been seen by her surgeon. Because of Dave's absence and Martin being unaware that Mrs. Sanders was in his care, this did not occur. Time passed, then Mrs. Sanders' condition suddenly deteriorated, with a rapid pulse and low blood pressure. The nurse tried to contact Dave but was unsuccessful and it was eventually established that Dave was on vacation. Martin was contacted and came at once. It was not difficult for Martin to determine that Mrs. Sanders was in septic shock and needed an immediate operation if her life was to be saved. In surgery, Martin found widespread severe infection called peritonitis, caused by a bowel perforation presumably sustained during the gall bladder operation. Because of the delay in the diagnosis, Mrs. Sanders had a very stormy post-operative course and required intensive treatment; she almost did not survive and it took her many months to recover.

When Dave returned from vacation, he was devastated to discover what had happened to Mrs. Sanders. Of course he was blamed for the entire incident. The immediate cause of the peritonitis was an injury to the bowel due to the cautery equipment. Dave believed the injury occurred during the time the picture disappeared from the monitor when the circulating nurse tripped over the cable. Multiple other factors contributed to this major adverse event.

ISSUES IN MINIMALLY INVASIVE SURGERY

Minimally Invasive Surgery (MIS), also referred to as minimal access surgery, endoscopic surgery, or keyhole surgery, is a relatively new surgical area. Surgery, the work of the surgeon's hand, has been revolutionized by the introduction of the endoscope, an instrument with a tiny video camera on the end, that enables surgeons to view inside a body cavity. Depending on which internal cavity is being viewed, the surgery is named accordingly; for example, laparoscopic for abdominal, thoracoscopic for chest, arthroscopic for joint surgery. Initially, endoscopes were used to see inside the body for exploratory and diagnostic purposes only. Eventually, surgeons were able to manipulate target tissues in the internal cavities to achieve surgical goals with specialized laparoscopic instruments. Thus, the purpose of such minimally invasive surgeries evolved from diagnostic to therapeutic. Although the focus of this discussion is primarily on laparoscopic procedures (see also Scott-Conner, 1999), many of the factors discussed also apply to other endoscopic surgical specialties.

The first laparoscopic cholecystectomy (gall bladder removal) was performed on a human patient in 1987 (Mouret, 1991; see also Reddick et al., 1989). Just over one decade later, almost all abdominal surgical procedures are performed laparoscopically. For such surgery, the patient requires general anesthetic, and as with Mrs. Sanders' case, the abdomen is insufflated with carbon dioxide. Small keyhole-size incisions are made for ports of entry of the camera and surgical instruments. These are inserted with the operative ends inside the abdominal cavity and the handles the surgeons use to control the instruments outside the patient's abdomen. Laparoscopic cholecystectomy has gained universal acceptance as the procedure of choice for gall bladder removal because of a high rate of success and rapid recovery in most cases. MIS procedures are used frequently for appendectomies, inguinal hernia repairs, and Nissen fundoplications, a procedure to alleviate severe heartburn. Compared to conventional open surgery, it is stated that laparoscopic operations reduce pain, suffering, and scarring, and shorten the patients' recovery time and hospital stays. It is likely that with further advances in technology and continuing patient demand, MIS will become an even more important and pervasive domain of surgery.

MIS involves highly complex technology. Such technologies have evolved often without controlled testing and evaluation prior to being introduced into the marketplace and the operating room. The complexity of the technology and the problems inherent in such complexity, particularly when the technology has not been subjected to controlled testing, have created an environment where errors and near misses occur, as was evident in the story of Mrs. Sanders' surgery. Increased vigilance is required of the surgeons because the consequences of problems in this complex technology fall square on them as the primary users of endoscopic technology in the operating room. Yet factors in the context in which the surgery is performed—for example, shortcomings in the environment where the surgeon operates such as cables and other clutter in the operating room—can affect performance and the outcome of the operation, ultimately compromising the well-being of the patient.

ERROR PROVOKING FACTORS

The evolution of endoscopic technologies and adoption of MIS procedures in general surgery has been rapid and pervasive; however, little research has been conducted to date on factors that affect the performance of surgeons using that technology (MacKenzie, Ibbotson, Cao, & Lomax, 1998). MIS is an extremely difficult, highly demanding, remote manipulation task. Skilled surgeons, however, make surgical tasks appear easy, although they often use inadequate or relatively primitive instruments for the tasks they are performing.

The story of Dave Gardner illustrates that there is no shortage of identifiable factors contributing to errors and potentially compromising patient safety in MIS (Cao et al., 1999; Ibbotson, MacKenzie, Cao, & Lomax, 1999). Some of the problems may seem unimportant; however, for any individual patient they could be very significant. These factors have a time frame. In general, problems are encountered more frequently early in the surgical procedures, in the transitions between different surgical steps and tasks, and with the insertion of new endoscopic instruments. Other factors are important to address to reduce the likelihood of error and enhance patient safety; many such factors were included in the story of Dave Gardner. Among those factors are instruments for surgical manipulation, viewing the surgical site, actions of the surgeon, equipment organization and layout, and communication and coordination in the operating room.

Instruments for Surgical Manipulation

Although the instruments for MIS are relatively primitive and have many limitations, skilled surgeons appear to be able to work with them. Figure 5.1 shows

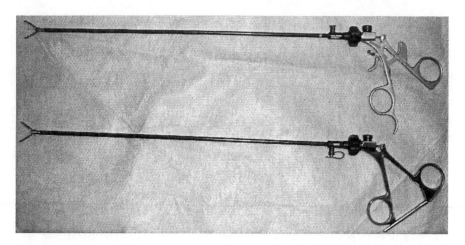

FIG. 5.1.   Two laparoscopic grasping tools, the bottom one with ratchet.

two reusable graspers used in laparoscopic surgery (Storz Endoscopy). The instruments are limited because they can be moved only in certain directions: they can be inserted and removed; moved at an angle about the fulcrum, the point of support at the entry port; rotated about a longitudinal axis as in turning the instrument inside the body cavity; and made to open and close. These limitations restrict the surgeons' movement of the instruments and frequently force awkward postures of the arms and shoulders, hence can influence the execution of the surgical procedure. Surgeons who perform MIS complain of fatigue; there are reports of repetitive strain injuries. In one instance, a surgeon had surgery to correct carpal tunnel syndrome in his preferred hand (MacKenzie et al., 1998).

The port or point of entry of the instrument into the abdomen acting as a fulcrum is important because at the entry point fulcrum, an instrument becomes a lever, which means small movements made by the surgeon on the outer end result in large movements of the end of the instrument in the body cavity. This makes delicate, precise movements of the working end of the instrument, the end that grasps and cuts inside the body (referred to as the end-effector), difficult (Patkin & Isabel, 1995).

Typically, one thinks of surgical instruments as reusable; however, reusable instruments can be difficult to clean and reassemble after cleaning. Lack of standardization of instruments from different manufacturers sometimes creates difficulties during the operation. This is evident in the story when Dave could not insert an instrument from one manufacturer into a cannula made by a different manufacturer. Loose working parts on the ends of the instruments such as laparoscopic graspers, an instrument with end-effectors that are expected to grasp tissue, can be ineffective. The surgeon may not be able to identify that problem until the instrument is removed from the abdominal cavity and visually examined, when the loose working parts become obvious.

Another significant problem that has not been solved yet is that reusable scissors become dull when used with cautery, as Dave discovered in conducting Mrs. Sanders' surgery. To reduce the likelihood of some of the problems with reusable instruments, disposable instruments are available. They have some characteristics that make them preferable to reusable instruments; however, the recurring cost of such throw-away instruments sometimes leads to their reuse to reduce cost.

Initial difficulties with the instrument handles, handles that can include buttons, switches, and dials to control the capabilities of the instrument, occur frequently when new instruments are introduced. For example, some rigid instruments can be rotated in the body cavity through the use of a rotary dial (similar to a volume control knob on a radio) on the surgeons' end of the instrument, but surgeons rarely use this dial because a hand is necessary to rotate the dial as the other holds the instrument and both of the surgeon's hands are actively occupied with instruments. Because surgeons cannot use the dial to rotate the instrument, they adopt awkward postures of their shoulders, wrists, and other parts of their bodies to move about the instrument. Such constraints imposed by the instrument lead to complaints by surgeons of local aches in the hand, wrist, or shoulders, as well as fatigue.

Cautery, also known as high-frequency electrosurgery, is a patient safety issue and source of errors in MIS. Cautery involves passing an electric current down the scissors or grasper to allow cutting of tissues, while controlling the bleeding of damaged blood vessels through the use of heat. Injury can occur to sites remote from the target tissues through tissue conduction by unintended contact, as in Mrs. Sanders' bowel perforation, as well as insulation breaks (Shimi, 1995; see also Voyles & Tucker, 1992). Even a slight break in the insulation of an MIS electrocautery instrument is serious. Electrodes without insulation can come into unintended contact with instruments that have intact active electrodes and activate them to conduct heat or induce the electric currents to surrounding instruments. Regardless of how it occurs, a break in the insulation provides the conditions for stray current to injure tissues.

The dissatisfaction of MIS surgeons with the suction and irrigation instrument stems from its lack of effectiveness when used to clear the operative field when bleeding obscures the video view. It is considerably more difficult to clear the field of blood using the suction and irrigation MIS instrument than in an open operation. At the end of a procedure, there are vital steps to avoid severe tissue damage—steps that underscore the importance of seeing the surgical site, which makes having the site clear of blood very important. It is imperative that the end of the instruments in the body cavity be viewed on the monitor during the final surgical step to ensure that all target tissues and organs held or in contact with the instruments are released prior to removal of the instruments. Otherwise, tissues might be torn when the instruments are removed, leading to complications.

Video Viewing of the Surgical Site

A clear video view of the surgical site inside the body cavity is critical; without that, the surgeon works blindly. Resolution or image detail is a crucial factor in correct perception (Cuschieri, 1995). The clarity of the image on the monitor that the surgeon views when performing an MIS procedure is significantly degraded compared to natural viewing. This is compounded by the fact that the field of view of the operative site displayed to the MIS surgeon is reduced compared to an open procedure. Such tunnel vision acts as a constraint on the surgeon and is another factor making MIS more difficult than open surgery. Luminance (brightness), chrominance (color), and depth perception as well as resolution are all important factors in the video image (Boppert, Deutsch, & Rattner, 1999).

Improvement in resolution will facilitate depth perception, which is important because the video monitor displays a flat, two-dimensional image. The lack of three-dimensional depiction of the operative site contributes to making MIS procedures difficult because the surgeon's actions must be coordinated with what is seen on the monitor. That is, the surgeon's hand movements on instrument handles outside of the body must coordinate with the endoscopic view of instrument end-effectors and target tissues inside the body.

Attempts to introduce 3-D systems into MIS have not met with success. Nonetheless, effective 3-D imaging would improve patient safety by making complex MIS tasks, such as suturing, easier (Crosthwaite, Chung, Dunkley, Shimi, & Cuschieri, 1995; Hanna, Shimi, & Cuschieri, 1998; MacKenzie, Graham, Cao, & Lomax, 1999).

The endoscopic surgeons' nightmare is to lose the picture of the surgical site on the video display because of a loose cable connection or unintentional disconnection. A more common occurrence is the clarity of the picture being severely compromised because the camera lens of the endoscope is covered with blood and body fluids, which necessitates frequent cleaning of the lens to remove the blood or fog. This can be done as Dave did in the story, by rubbing the lens against a target tissue inside the body, or removing the endoscope for cleaning then reinserting it. Surgeons can be frustrated by problems with image clarity, focus, color, and contrast on the video monitors; however, the limited field of view is one of the major limitations of endoscopic video imaging, as noted in the story.

To obtain both the necessary detail and a view of anatomical context of the surgical site, it is necessary for the surgeons to continually zoom the lens in and out of the MIS viewing target area. Zooming the lens in the target area typically provides magnification of two to three times, hence additional detail vital for the surgeon's clear, direct view of the trocar insertion and operative sites. The surgeon must see where sharp trocars will be inserted, and where end-effectors will be positioned, to avoid injury. Incidents have occurred where the aorta was punctured by insertion of the first trocar or injured in other ways. Inserted instruments in active use must always be in view. Instruments not centered and observed by the surgeon in the field of view have punctured or perforated vessels and organs such as the bile duct, bowel, liver, and esophagus (Cuschieri, 1995). Such focus on detail, although vital in performing the procedure, sacrifices a larger view of the anatomical context of the target area because of the tunnel vision imposed by the camera lens.

Actions of Surgeons

Frequently the foot pedals activating the cautery equipment are confused with pedals for other instruments such as the pedal for scissors that can be mistaken for the pedal for the harmonic scalpel. Such instruments can become activated by someone stepping on a pedal. Inadvertent activation of the cautery is a danger because the surgeon would not be aware it was hot and it could burn by contacting tissues or organs. An instrument that is hot also could ignite the paper drapes covering the patient with disastrous results.

On occasions, surgeons can be so immersed in the procedure that their roles as primary surgeon (manipulating instruments) or assisting surgeon (controlling camera) are confused. For example, a surgeon can move his or her hand and be surprised that the view on the monitor does not change correspondingly; the surgeon actually is moving the grasper, not the camera. This speaks to the intense concentration, focused attention, and the complexity of the coordination required between what the surgeons see on the video monitor and how their hands control the end-effectors of instruments in the body cavity. This creates a sense of presence experienced by the surgeon who is totally immersed in the video-endoscopic environment to perform surgical tasks.

Equipment Organization and Layout
in the Operating Room

Many independent, isolated pieces of equipment reside in the OR. How they are organized within that space is important for reducing the likelihood of error. Placement of equipment that hinders movement or restricts vision can create ongoing frustration during the procedure. Monitors, intravenous lines, cautery equipment, and irrigation and suction devices can be difficult to access and at the same time restrict activity. The large number of cables from independent pieces of equipment makes moving around difficult in a crowded operating room. Other equipment, carts, or drapes placed by the anesthesiologist over the patient can obscure the view of the video monitor for the primary or assisting surgeons.

Electrical interference (cross talk) between the cables for cautery and those for the video camera can affect the clarity of the monitor display. Attempts to avoid this through layout of the equipment as an integrated operating room is a concept that is being actively pursued by various researchers (Frank, Hanna, & Cuschieri, 1997; Schurr & Buess, 1995) and companies. In 2003, integrated ORs are being installed in many large academic hospitals. A factor that can thwart such integration is the lack of standardization in equipment made by different manufacturers (Herron, Gagner, Kenyon, & Swanstrom, 2001).

Surgical technologies need to be integrated, rather than functioning as separate, isolated pieces of equipment (Herron, Gagner, Kenyon, & Swanstrom, 2001; Schurr & Buess, 1995). This is especially true for the location for manipulating in the operative space and the endoscopic view of that space. The primary surgeon often views the image of the operative field at nearly a right angle from where the instruments are being manipulated. This is illustrated in Fig. 5.2,

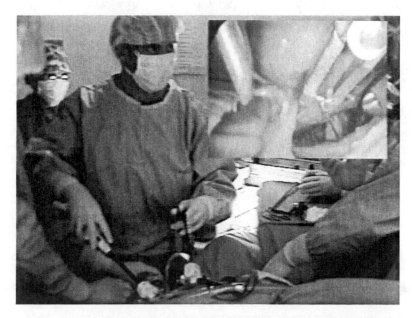

FIG. 5.2. One frame of our split-screen videotape of laparoscopic surgery (faces digitally modified to ensure anonymity). The inset shows the endoscopic camera's view.

which shows a screen from a research video in which the gaze of the primary surgeon is directed to the monitor that is away from the physical location of the instruments and the patient's abdomen—an assisting surgeon, a surgical resident, and two nurses are in the background. The insert in Fig. 5.2 is the image of the patient's abdomen provided by the video-endoscopic camera.

Technologies that superimpose the video image on the actual external location of the operative site, thus decreasing the complexity of remote manipulation, are a high priority (MacKenzie et al., 1999; Mandryk & MacKenzie, 1999). This would allow the surgeons to view the operating site in a straight line with where their hands are manipulating the instruments, which facilitates hand–eye coordination.

Communication and Coordination in the Operating Room

A great deal of noise is generated by equipment, the intercom, paging systems, and conversation in the operating rooms of teaching hospitals. Because of this, communication among the surgical staff (surgeons, residents, anesthesiologists, and nurses) may not be heard clearly, resulting in miscommunication. In addition, the similar sound emitted by various devices as well as pagers in an operating room can be confusing, as illustrated by Dave Gardner's confusing the beep of his pager with that of a cautery device pedal alarm.

CONCLUDING COMMENTS

The story of Dave Gardner and the laparoscopic cholecystectomy he performed on Mrs. Sanders illustrates how a number of factors that are beyond the control of the care provider in the context in which care is delivered, in this instance the context for performing MIS, contributed to if not provoked error. Some of the factors identified in the story can have life-threatening consequences either singly or as part of a cascade of events that lead to an adverse outcome. An example of the latter is Mrs. Sanders' perforated bowel that was the outcome of a number of factors: the clutter in the operating room that set the stage for Mary Monroe, the circulating nurse in the story, to trip over the video monitor cable, causing the picture of the surgical site to be lost, which kept Dave from seeing the spark that flew to Mrs. Sanders' bowel and perforated it. Even if the image of the surgical site had not been lost, the perforation of Mrs. Sanders' bowel might have been outside Dave's line of sight given the tunnel vision created by the lens.

Additional factors may contribute to patient morbidity (make the patient sicker) or to an iatrogenic problem (a problem that is caused by the treatment the patient receives, as in Mrs. Sanders' perforated bowel). Other pervasive factors that can contribute to error and an adverse outcome are aspects of the endoscopic technologies and their lack of integration. These factors in the systems that comprise the context of care adversely affect the ease, efficiency, and effectiveness, hence the safety, of the surgeon's work. They also have an economic significance because the delays resulting from coping with these factors prolong the time the patient is in the operating room and significantly increase costs both monetary and in terms of safety because a fatigued or frustrated surgeon is more likely to be involved in an error during endoscopic surgery than one who is rested and whose work environment is supportive of the tasks to be performed when conducting that surgery (Joice, Hanna, & Cuschieri, 1998).

The surgeon using MIS technologies is working within the larger operating room team in that complex setting. The story of Dave Gardner and research show that many factors in the context of care—the instruments, the clutter, and the condition of the patient such as the extreme inflammation of Mrs. Sanders' gall bladder—have the potential to cause errors and compromise safety. To enhance patient safety, attention must be paid to these factors. To reduce the likelihood of incidents and adverse outcomes, it is necessary to determine where, how, when, and most importantly *why* errors occur. Factors that contribute to the errors must be identified and strategies for rectifying them be devised and implemented, thus enhancing patient safety.

ACKNOWLEDGMENTS

Observational research in hospital operating rooms was funded by the British Columbia Health Research Foundation, now the Michael Smith Foundation for Health Research in British Columbia, Canada. We thank all surgical staff and especially the patients for their cooperation and participation. Preparation of this chapter was supported in part by funds from Canada's Networks of Centre of Excellence, Institute for Robotics and Intelligent Systems (IRIS3), Intelligent Tools for Health Care Project, to C. L. MacKenzie at Simon Fraser University.

REFERENCES

Boppert, S. A., Deutsch, T. F., & Rattner, D. W. (1999). Optical imaging technology in minimally invasive surgery. *Surgical Endoscopy, 13,* 718–722.

Cao, C. G. L., MacKenzie, C. L., Ibbotson, J. A., Turner, L. J., Blair, N. P., & Nagy, A. G. (1999). Hierarchical decomposition of laparoscopic procedures. In J. D. Westwood, H. M. Hoffman, R. A. Robb, & D. Stredney (Eds.), *Medicine meets virtual reality. The convergence of physical and informational technologies: Options for a new era in healthcare. (MMVR:7)* (pp. 83–89). Amsterdam: IOS Press.

Crosthwaite, G., Chung, T., Dunkley, P., Shimi, S., & Cuschieri, A. (1995). Comparison of direct vision and electronic 2- and 3-D display systems on surgical task efficiency in endoscopic surgery. *Annals of Surgery, 82,* 849–851.

Cuschieri, A. (1995). Visual displays and visual perception in minimal access surgery. *Seminars in Laparoscopic Surgery, 2*(3), 209–214.

Frank, T. G., Hanna, G. B., & Cuschieri, A. (1997). Technological aspects of minimal access surgery. *Proceedings of the Institute of Mechanical Engineers. Part H—Journal of Engineering in Medicine, 211*(2), 129–144.

Hanna, G. B., Shimi, S. M., & Cuschieri, A. (1998). Randomized study of influence of two-dimensional versus three-dimensional imaging on performance of laparoscopic cholecystectomy. *The Lancet, 351,* 248–251.

Herron, D. M., Gagner, M., Kenyon, T. M., & Swanstrom, L. L. (2001). The minimally invasive surgery suite enters the 21st century. *Surgical Endoscopy, 15,* 415–422.

Ibbotson, J. A., MacKenzie, C. L., Cao, C. G. L., & Lomax, A. J. (1999). Gaze patterns in laparoscopic surgery. In J. D. Westwood, H. M. Hoffman, R. A. Robb, & D. Stredney (Eds.), *Medicine meets virtual reality. The convergence of physical and informational technologies: Options for a new era in healthcare. (MMVR:7)* (pp. 154–160). Amsterdam: IOS Press.

Joice, P., Hanna, G. B., & Cuschieri, A. (1998). Errors enacted during endoscopic surgery—a human reliability analysis. *Applied Ergonomics, 29,* 409–414.

MacKenzie, C. L., Graham, E. D., Cao, C. G. L., & Lomax, A. J. (1999). Virtual hand laboratory meets endoscopic surgery. In J. D. Westwood, H. M. Hoffman, R. A. Robb, & D. Stredney (Eds.), *Medicine meets virtual reality. The convergence of physical and informational technologies: Options for a new era in healthcare. (MMVR:7)* (pp. 212–218). Amsterdam: IOS Press.

MacKenzie, C. L., Ibbotson, J. A., Cao, C. G. L., & Lomax, A. J. (1998). Intelligent instruments for minimally invasive surgery: Safety and error issues. In A. L. Scheffler & L. A. Zipperer (Eds.), *Proceedings of enhancing patient safety and reducing errors in health care* (pp. 226–229). Chicago: National Patient Safety Foundation.

Mandryk, R. L., & MacKenzie, C. L. (1999). Superimposing display space on workspace in the context of endoscopic surgery. *Association for Computing Machinery Computer–Human Interaction CHI99 Extended Abstracts, Association for Computing Machinery Press,* 284–285.

Mouret, P. (1991). From the first laparoscopic cholecystectomy to the frontiers of laparoscopic surgery; the future perspective. *Digestive Surgery, 8,* 12–15.

Patkin, M., & Isabel, L. (1995). Ergonomics, engineering and surgery of endosurgical dissection. *Journal of the Royal College of Surgeons of Edinburgh, 40*(2), 120–132.

Reddick, E. J., Olsen, D. O., Daniell, J. F., Saye, W. B., Muller, W., & Holback, M. (1989). Laparoscopic laser cholecystectomy. *Laser Medical and Surgical News, 7,* 38–40.

Schurr, M. O., & Buess, G. (1995). OREST II: Ergonomic workplace and systems platform for endoscopic technologies. *Endoscopic Surgery, 3,* 193–198.

Scott-Conner, C. E. H. (Ed.). (1999). *SAGES (Society of American Gastrointestinal and Endoscopic Surgery) Manual: Fundamentals of Laparoscopy and GI Endoscopy.* New York: Springer-Verlag.

Shimi, S. H. (1995). Dissection techniques in laparoscopic surgery. *Journal of the Royal College of Surgeons of Edinburgh, 40,* 249–259.

Voyles, C. R., & Tucker, R. D. (1992). Education and engineering solutions for potential problems with laparoscopic monopolar electrosurgery. *American Journal of Surgery, 166*(4), 440–441.

6 The Laparoscopic Surgeon's Posture

Ulrich Matern

University Hospital of Tübingen, Germany

SURGEON, DR. ARTHUR

Dr. Arthur is a young, talented surgeon. He has successfully performed many operations, most of them as traditional open surgery. In this method of performing surgery, the abdominal wall of the patient is opened by an incision large enough to view the surgical field and adjacent organs and insert a hand into the abdominal cavity to directly touch and feel the organs. Today Dr. Arthur is scheduled to perform laparoscopic surgery, a relatively new type of surgery, in which several small incisions are made in the abdomen, through which instruments with long shafts are inserted to perform the surgery. The shafts are long to accommodate the distance from the outside of the patient's abdomen to the internal organs. A tiny video optic inserted into one of the incisions sends images of parts of the surgical field to an external monitor. The surgeon uses the images on the monitor to guide the movement of the instruments inside the abdominal cavity.

Dr. Arthur is to use the laparoscopic technique to perform a gall bladder dissection (removal) in Mrs. Fenchurch, a corpulent 42-year-old woman with a gall bladder filled with stones. He, like other surgeons, feels a little uncomfortable about this type of surgery because of the way he has to maneuver the long instruments. He compares using these instruments to eating Chinese food with chopsticks. Nevertheless, he has performed many operations like this one. Laparoscopic surgery is popular with patients because of the improved cosmetic results of no large scar and less postoperative pain compared to open proce-

dures. From the surgeon's point of view, this method has some disadvantages due to the technical equipment.

When Dr. Arthur enters the operating room (OR) in the morning, he finds that his colleagues Dr. Ford, Dr. Zaphod, and the nurses have positioned Mrs. Fenchurch on the operating table. She is in deep anesthesia; her arms are set at about 90° as if on a cross. Her body is covered with green sterile paper drapes reaching to the floor with only the upper two thirds of her abdomen visible. Dr. Ford and Dr. Zaphod are standing next to Mrs. Fenchurch, ready to assist Dr. Arthur. Next to her outstretched right arm stands a tall rack with several devices, the technical equipment for laparoscopic surgery. On the top of the rack is the video monitor on which Dr. Arthur views his work. As he is not very tall, only 5 feet 6 inches, it is necessary for him to look up to the monitor to follow the procedure. Next to the patient's feet Mrs. Trillian, the nurse, has positioned a table with the surgical instruments they will need for the operation—scalpels, scissors, and forceps. Many tubes and cables connect these surgical instruments with various devices in the rack such as the light source for illuminating the interior of the abdominal cavity so the video can work and the generator for electrocautery to cut tissue and seal off bleeding vessels with heat.

In case there is a problem with the laparoscopic procedure, instruments for open surgery are on a table next to several laparoscopic instruments. Unlike the instruments for open surgery, the shafts of the laparoscopic instruments are as long as Dr. Arthur's forearm, and thin. The diameter is comparable to that of a pencil. At one end of these instruments are tiny effectors to cut or grasp tissue. On the other end, the instruments have different types of handles such as a handle similar to that of a pair of scissors or a shank handle. The handles are angled in different degrees with respect to the shaft of the instrument. Next to those instruments are the trocars, tubes with valves through which the instruments are inserted into the abdomen of the patient. The abdomen is infused or filled with carbon dioxide gas to clear a space between the abdominal wall and the organs; space is needed to move the instruments and the camera to visualize the operation. The valves in the trocars keep the gas from escaping when changing instruments, hence keeping the abdomen infused.

Dr. Arthur reaches the left side of the patient by climbing over cables and tubes to the instruments and squeezes himself between the instrument table and Dr. Ford. Dr. Arthur is a little corpulent himself and feels quite crowded at the operating table when he is surrounded by all the technical equipment and the operating staff. Dr. Arthur asks a nurse to lower the operating table to position the patient's abdominal wall at the level of his hip so he can manipulate the instruments. He then inserts the needle through the abdominal wall and after performing the usual security tests to make certain that the needle is in its correct position, connects it with the tube leading to the device to insufflate gas into the abdomen. The gas expands Mrs. Fenchurch's abdominal cavity, which lifts her abdominal wall a couple of inches, raising Dr. Arthur's work area. He again asks that the table be lowered so he can work in an upright position without standing on tiptoe.

The surgery begins when Dr. Arthur uses the scalpel to cut four small incisions into Mrs. Fenchurch's abdominal skin. He pushes the first trocar through the small incision in the abdominal wall at the patient's belly button after the first needle was extracted. The gas tube is connected to that trocar for continuous gas insufflation. He then inserts an optic as long as the instrument's shaft through the trocar to take pictures of the inside of the abdomen. A small camera is attached to the end of the optic outside the patient. The camera is connected to the light source and the video terminal by two cables. Dr. Ford manages the camera to make certain that Dr. Arthur can see on the monitor what he is doing inside Mrs. Fenchurch's abdomen. Dr. Arthur wants to improve his view of the surgical field by lowering the position of the monitor; however, the monitor can only be moved slightly to the side. He places the final trocars in the abdominal wall and inserts the long-shafted instruments into them.

Dr. Zaphod holds the instrument for grasping and holding the gall bladder. Each of the two instruments Dr. Arthur holds has a different type of handle. With his left hand, he is manipulating a pair of forceps with a ring handle angled to the instrument at about 90°; it is necessary to grasp that handle from below. With his right hand, he holds an instrument for electrocautery with a pencil-like handle. His right arm is elevated and his left arm is lowered, putting his shoulder in an inclined position with his backbone bent to the right.

Dr. Arthur needs an electrocautery instrument for blood control and tissue dissection that is connected by a cable to the power source. He is positioned to use his right foot to activate a foot switch that turns the power to that instrument on and off. Next to that switch is a foot switch to control the rinsing and suctioning instrument that is used when there is bleeding. The height of Mrs. Fenchurch's expanded abdomen with respect to Dr. Arthur's arms makes it necessary for him to be standing on his tiptoes to use the electrocautery instrument while simultaneously coordinating the various instruments in his and his assistant's hands.

The movement of the members of the operating team is hindered by the many cables and tubes in the vicinity of the operating table. It is nearly impossible for Dr. Arthur to find a comfortable position for optimal manipulation of the instruments. In addition, he wishes for a better view of the monitor that is positioned far away and now is partially obscured by Dr. Zaphod so he leans forward in an attempt to see. He seeks to solve some of the problems by asking that the operating table be lowered again and is told the table already is at its lowest position. To obtain the necessary height with respect to Mrs. Fenchurch's abdomen, Dr. Arthur decides to stand on a stool-like platform. That platform is so small that he has just enough space for his feet and the foot switch for elec- trocautery. The lack of space makes it necessary that Dr. Ford operates the other foot switch. Dr. Arthur is grateful that additional devices controlled by foot switches, such as an ultrasound dissector or an argon beamer, are not needed in this simple routine case.

As is common for many surgeons, Dr. Arthur remembers the uncomfortable feeling of "What will happen next?" that he experienced when he entered the OR this morning. He wonders if problems will arise with the insufflating gas, the video system, electric power, or the pain, cramps, and fatigue he experiences in his arms and backbone after working in the nearly unbearable position that is necessary for laparoscopic surgery. For the next half hour, the OR team con- centrates and works quite well without any problems. Suddenly a small bleed occurs. It is not dramatic—only a small incident. Dr. Arthur inserts the suction and irrigation instrument into the abdominal cavity to clean the blood from the organs so he will have a clear image of what is happening and to coagulate the vessel with his electrocautery instrument.

Dr. Ford presses the foot switch for suction. To do this, he has to stand on one foot which causes the camera to move a little to the side. This disturbs Dr. Arthur's view of the bleeding. Nevertheless, he works to coagulate the blood ves- sel with the long shafted electrocautery instrument in his right hand and perform suctioning with the instrument in his left hand. As Dr. Arthur reaches with his right foot to activate the electric instrument, the switch falls off the platform and he loses his balance, which moves the electrocautery instrument. It scratches the surface of the patient's liver, causing heavy bleeding.

ADVERSE EVENTS WAITING TO HAPPEN

Although this story is fiction, every incident in it occurs regularly during laparo- scopic surgery. The importance of laparoscopic procedures in visceral surgery has constantly increased in the last 10 years. Laparoscopic removal of the gall bladder has become the gold standard. The number of laparoscopic surgeries is rising; however, there still are technical problems and disadvantages in the pro- cedure that need further research.

Procedural Constraints

In laparoscopic surgical procedures, the surgeon loses direct contact with the surgical site. Rather than seeing the entire surgical field including adjacent organs, the surgeon's vision is restricted to the point of surgery, and the view depends on the angle of the camera. The surgeon does not have the tactile feed-back of open surgery due to the length of the shaft of the surgical instruments. In addition, the freedom of movement of the video camera and the long-shafted instruments is limited because they are fixed in the abdominal wall. This forces the surgeon into unnatural and uncomfortable body postures that can affect the outcome of the operation. The problems caused by the posture the surgeon must assume in actually performing laparoscopic surgery become apparent when the ideal body posture for laparoscopic surgery is considered.

Ideal Body Posture in Laparoscopic Surgery.   The person is standing upright. The head is bent forward at the angle of a slight nod (Berguer, 1999) or preferably in varying positions. Increased angling of the head and neck over a long period of time should be avoided because that results in tension and pain of the neck muscles. The most favorable angle of the elbow is that for industrial employees, 90° to 120°. The arms can be held at this range of angles for a long period of time (Bullinger, 1994). The horizontal position of the forearm is rec-ommended for laparoscopic surgery (Laparoscopic Surgery Update, 1997). The favorable working angle between two instruments for stitching and knotting as in suturing in a laparoscopic procedure is 60° (Hanna, Shimi, & Cuschieri, 1997). This angle conforms to a slightly inward-rotated, comfortable position of the arm. The wrist should have a slightly extended position (Matern & Waller, 1999). The fingers are bent slightly as in the natural position of the hand (Matern & Waller, 1999). From this position, any possible grip can be performed quickly and easily (Bullinger, 1979) as illustrated in Fig. 6.1 and Fig. 6.2.

Positions other than these, especially when they are static, lead to rapid fatigue, muscle pain, and cramps (Grandjean, 1982). This can affect the sur-geon's performance and possibly result in an adverse event. Several factors inherent in laparoscopic surgery induce postures that are far from the ideal.

Factors in Laparoscopic Surgery That Determine the Posture of the Surgeons

When performing laparoscopic procedures, factors inherent to that type of sur-gery constrain not only the surgeons' posture but also their view of the surgical site. Those factors can contribute to error and subsequent adverse outcomes.

Position of the Monitor.   Observing the abdominal cavity via a video image on the monitor is of tantamount importance to the surgeon. The image of the surgical site must be seen to determine the placement of the surgical instru-ments. Thus, the position of the monitor in large part dictates the body posture of the surgeon. This is illustrated in the story when Dr. Arthur, while conducting

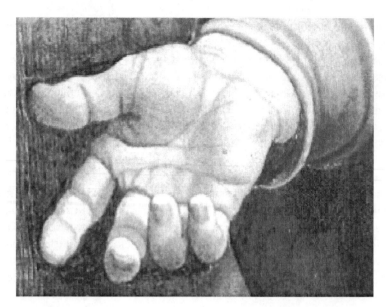

FIG. 6.1. Optimal position of the hand (Ezechiel, Michelangelo, Sistine Chapel, Rome, 1516).

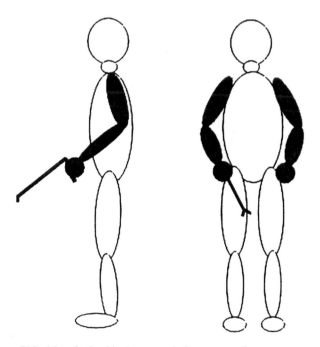

FIG. 6.2. Optimal body posture in laparoscopy for surgeons.

surgery, has to lean forward to see the monitor that is partially blocked by Dr. Zaphod.

The small area around the patient in the OR is not sufficient to move the rack to improve visibility of the monitor to ease the posture of the surgeon. The height of the monitor on the rack cannot be adjusted to accommodate the height of the surgeon. Tall surgeons have a horizontal view of the monitor. Small surgeons, many of whom are women, have to look up to view the monitor. Such posture is counter to the recommended neck position and leads to neck pain. In addition, the vertical level view of the image on the monitor is different from the position of the surgeon's hands at the surgical site.

The problem also exists in surgery of the upper abdomen. For this surgical location, the monitor should be positioned in the area of the head of the patient; however, that rarely occurs because the anesthetist needs that space. Such disparities of location of the monitor with respect to the hands of the surgeon can lead to difficulties in hand–eye coordination (Berguer, 1999; Griesel, 1995; Hanna et al., 1997). Contorted working positions compromise the surgeon's direct control of happenings outside the patient's abdominal wall. Shafts of instruments may collide, cables and tubes become entangled, and the discovery of leaking valves in trocars delayed. The latter problem causes reduction of the space for viewing and the movement of instruments in the abdominal cavity. This also can impact the surgeon's performance. In addition to the position of the monitor, the body posture of the surgeon is determined by the design of the laparoscopic surgical instruments.

Handle Shape of the Surgical Instruments.   Although the length of the shaft is fairly consistent across laparoscopic surgical instruments, various types of handles are available. The most common are ring handles similar to those on scissors and shank handles that are commonly used on pruning shears. These handles are available in angled or axial orientation in relation to the shaft of the instrument. Either handle can be used with one hand to operate the two functions of the instrument: opening and closing the effector, and rotating the effector. Additional functions such as angling the shaft can only be performed with two hands, which necessitates interrupting the procedure while the surgeon gets off the second instrument.

The position of the hand varies according to the type of handle. Axial handles are held with an extreme wrist deviation in the direction to the small finger to position the instrument in the direction of the patient (see Fig. 6.3). This deviation may lead to increased fatigue, pain, and cramps (Grandjean, 1982). Angled ring handles require the opposite wrist movement in the direction to the thumb to keep the instrument in the extension of the forearm's axis. In both handle types, a rotation of the tip of the instruments cannot be performed solely by

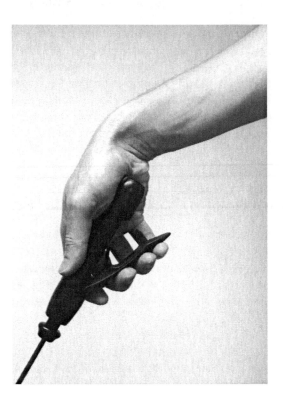

FIG. 6.3. The deviation of the wrist in the direction to the little finger when using the axial handle leads to fatigue, pain, and cramps.

turning the hand because the instrument's axis is not a direct extension of the forearm. For a simple rotation of the instrument's tip, both handle types require a large-scale movement of the entire arm from the shoulder. As the space is limited in the operating table area, a large movement is not always possible. Such movements may be complicated by the cables and tubes from the instruments; a large movement by the surgeon might change the position of other instruments in the abdominal cavity resulting in dangerous injuries.

A mixture of types of handles can be error-provoking because an instrument with an axial handle is held from above whereas the other instrument with the angled handle is held from below. Grasping the instruments in those ways leads to contorted body posture of the surgeon. Elevating one shoulder and sinking the other, as is necessary to use instruments with differing handles, leads to an asymmetric, totally unnatural posture.

Foot Controls. In contrast to open surgery in which the patient's abdomen is opened with a long incision that enables the assistants and surgeon to work with their hands in the abdominal cavity, in laparoscopic surgery the assistance of the OR team is limited to static functions of holding instruments and managing the camera. The dissection, the cutting and removal, as well as the sucking and rinsing activities are primarily performed by the surgeon. To accomplish this, it is necessary for the surgeon not only to hold and position the instruments, but also to simultaneously operate the foot switches for functions such as sucking and rinsing, electric cutting and coagulation, and if necessary activating additional instruments such as the ultrasonic scalpel and ultrasound dissector, and argon beamer—special devices for dissection and coagulation. Only foot switches are available for most of these instruments.

The number of foot switches limits the space for feet under the operating table. Often there is not enough space for the foot switches on the small platforms needed to compensate for the different heights of surgeons. To use the switches, the surgeon may have to perform his precise surgical movements while standing on one foot. Sometimes it is necessary for an assistant to operate one or more of the foot switches, as was done by Dr. Ford in the story. This creates a physical strain and requires immense concentration to avoid incorrect use of the instruments and switches during the course of the operation. These are conditions that provoke errors by the most competent and conscientious surgeon—errors that are beyond the control of the surgeon, as illustrated in the story.

Position of the Surgeon's Hands Relative to the Surgical Site.   Because of the length of the shaft of laparoscopic instruments and their being fixed in the abdominal wall of the patient, the position of the surgeon with respect to the prone patient on the operating table determines the possible variations in the surgeon's arm movements. In surgery of the upper abdomen, the surgeon may be positioned to the right or left of the patient or between the patient's straddled legs as illustrated in Fig. 6.4. The lateral and frontal position of the surgeon relative to the patient determines great differences in the arm movements necessary to perform the procedure. In the lateral position, more extreme arm movements are required to use the laparoscopic instruments to perform the surgical tasks (Eichenlaub, 1997).

Height of the Operating Table.   Adjustability of operating tables was discussed for a hundred years when only open surgery was performed (De Quervain, 1906, 1909). This is particularly important in laparoscopic surgery in which, for the surgeon to be best able to perform the procedure, the position of the operating table must be such that the abdominal wall of the patient is at the height of the upper third of the surgeon's thigh (Laparoscopic Surgery Update, 1997; Matern, Waller, Giebmeyer, Rückauer, & Farthmann, 2001).

The lowest adjustable surface of recently manufactured operating tables is approximately the height of a standard desk (Maquet, 1997), which is sufficient for open surgery. Only in rare cases do surgeons wish to adjust the table height

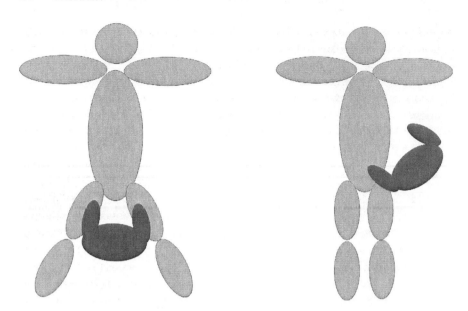

FIG. 6.4.   For operations of the upper abdomen, the surgeon may station himself or herself laterally to the patient or frontally, between the patient's legs.

lower than that for comfortable body posture during open surgery. Laparoscopic
surgery is a different situation.

At the beginning of a laparoscopic procedure when the trocars are introduced
into the abdominal wall, and at its conclusion when the wounds are closed, open
surgical techniques with short instruments such as normal surgical scissors are
used. Therefore, the operating table has to be relatively high for the surgeon to
work in an upright, standing posture. When the laparoscopic part of the surgery
begins, it is necessary to lower the table significantly. Due to the limited adjustability of the table, however, it cannot be lowered to the optimal position for a small
or medium height surgeon such as a woman to perform the necessary precise procedures in a noncontorted, relaxed posture (Matern, 1998; Matern et al., 2001).

To compensate for the difference in height between the patient on the too-
high operating table and the height to work in adequate posture, the surgeon has
two possibilities. The procedure can be performed with arms elevated to the
shoulder (see Fig. 6.5). This not only is very fatiguing (Grandjean, 1982) and
may cause long-lasting shoulder pains for the surgeon, but also such posture
changes the angle between operating tool and forearm, which can only be bal-
anced by excessive bending of the wrist. The resulting fatigue and pain in the
arm makes fine work such as suturing using the long-shafted instruments very
difficult.

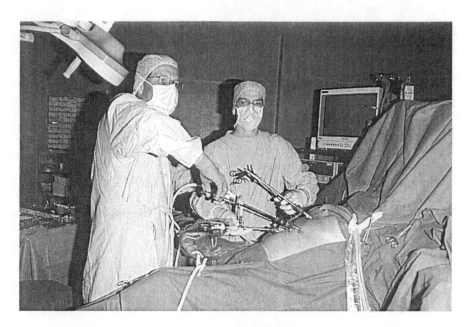

FIG. 6.5.   Surgeon performing dissection with elevated arms, as the patient is positioned too high.

The second possibility is for the surgeon to gain height by standing on a small platform. Usually there are only a few different-sized small platforms available, so the ideal position can rarely be achieved. The limited space for the feet of the surgeon on the platform is further restricted by foot switches for electrocautery instruments and the device that suctions fluids from the surgical site and irrigates the area with solutions. Often, foot switches for additional devices are placed on the platform, crowding the space so that a switch falls off (Matern, 1998; see Fig. 6.6). This is a dangerous, error-provoking situation because the surgeon can become unbalanced and injure the patient with an uncontrolled movement of an instrument, as illustrated in the story. In addition, the surgeon or members of the operating team may be injured when falling off the platform.

CONCLUSION

In laparoscopy, the surgeon performs distinct, minute movements of the instrument's tip in the abdominal cavity of the patient. To do this with the long-shafted instruments, it is sometimes necessary to make large arm movements. Imagine the working positions of a surgeon performing laparoscopic procedures standing on a small platform with one foot between several foot switches, back bent, one

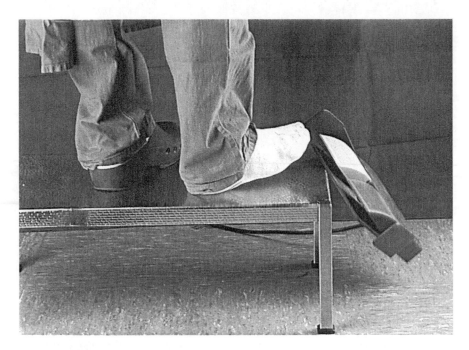

FIG. 6.6.   Smaller surgeon has to climb a foot step to achieve the required distance from the patient. The foot switches may slide away or fall from the step.

shoulder and arm lowered in a tense position to hold an organ with a forceps instrument while the other upturned arm conducts large movements, the wrists extremely angled and the fingers around the handle of an instrument to perform superfine dissection cuts in a sensitive region inside the patient. During this maneuver, the surgeon's head moves forward in an unnatural way to look in another direction at the monitor to observe the impact of these actions in the abdominal cavity of the patient.

Laparoscopic procedures usually take more time than open surgery. Because of the time involved, it is even more important for surgeons to work in a favorable posture. If the excessive fatigue resulting from postures necessary to compensate for operating room equipment that is inappropriate for laparoscopic surgery, such as a too-high operating table, could be avoided, then the surgeon and the patient would both benefit. The benefit to the patient not only is during the surgery, but also to those patients the surgeon cares for postoperatively. The fatigue and nervousness from the postural strain experienced during the surgical procedure can compromise the ability of the surgeon to deal with patient's postoperative issues. The impact of the surgeons' skills and talents being compromised by the equipment available to perform laparoscopic surgery reaches beyond the surgeons themselves and their patients.

Because of the shrinking resources for health care, it is extremely important to efficiently utilize available health care personnel. Hospital staffs have been and will continue to be reduced for cost savings. This is occurring as the number of elderly patients and their concomitant need for health care increases. To meet this as well as the other ongoing health care needs of the population, the workload of surgeons and other health care providers will increase. There is a limit to how much people can do, so they must work smarter.

Why do the conditions in which health care is provided often necessitate nearly superhuman effort to provide quality care? Surgeons, hospital administrators, and industry miss significant opportunities to learn to work smarter when they ignore knowledge and insight gained in other domains. It is imperative that this be overcome and that the lessons learned from others be applied to aspects of health care such as the laparoscopic surgery equipment and the OR environment to make the working conditions of surgeons amenable to their physiological and postural needs and by doing so reducing the likelihood of error.

Thanks to Dr. Arthur's experienced hands, Mrs. Fenchurch's gall bladder surgery had a happy ending. After taking a deep breath and reorganizing the instruments and foot switches, Dr. Arthur and his assistants regained their psychological balance and finally controlled the bleeding from the electrocautery instrument touching Mrs. Fenchurch's liver and finished the operation safely. Although she needed blood transfusions, Mrs. Fenchurch recovered well. Dr. Arthur, however, has chronic shoulder, neck, and back pain.

REFERENCES

Berguer, R. (1999). Surgery and ergonomics. *Archives of Surgery, 134,* 1011–1016.

Bullinger, H. J. (1979). *Ergonomische Arbeitsmittelgestaltung I—Systematik [Ergonomic workplace design I—Systematic].* Editor: Bundesanstalt für Arbeitsschutz und Unfallforschung Dortmund. Forschungsbericht 196. Wirtschaft NW.

Bullinger, H. J. (1994). *Ergonomie: Produkt und Arbeitsplatzgestaltung [Ergonomy: Product and workplace design].* Stuttgart: Teubner.

De Quervain, F. (1906). Zur Operationstischfrage [Question to operating table]. *Zentralblatt Chirurgie, 11,* 321–323.

De Quervain, F. (1909). Weiteres zur Operationstischfrage [More about operating tables]. *Zentralblatt Chirurgie, 19,* 686–688.

Eichenlaub, M. (1997). *Ergonomie von Handgriffen laparoskopischer Instrumente: eine experimentelle Studie [Ergonomics of handles for laparoscopic instruments: An experimental study].* Dissertation, Univ.-Hospital Freiburg, Germany.

Grandjean, E. (1982). Ergonomie in der Praxis [Ergonomics in practice]. *Schriftreihe Arbeitswissenschaft des Arbeitgeberverbandes der Metallindustrie.* Köln.

Griesel, R. (1995). Apparative Ausrüstung und Instrumente in der minimal invasiven Chirurgie. In A. Pier & E. Schippers, *Minimal Invasive Chirurgie: Grundlagen, Techniken, Ergebnisse, Trends* [*Devices and instruments for minimally invasive surgery*] (pp. 72–75). Thieme, Stuttgart New York.

Hanna, G. B., Shimi, S., & Cuschieri, A. (1997). Influence of direction of view, target-to-endoscope distance, and manipulation angle on endoscopic knot tying. *British Journal of Surgery, 84,* 1460–1464.

Laparoscopic Surgery Update. (1997). Reduce fatigue and discomfort: Tips to improve operating room setup. *Laparoscopic Surgery Update, 5,* 97–100.

Maquet, Inc. (1997). OP-Tisch-System: Alphamaquet 1150. *Product Information 8.* Rastatt, Germany: Author.

Matern, U. (1998). Ergonomische Aspekte der laparoskopischen Chirurgie [Ergonomic aspects of laparoscopic surgery]. *Sichere Arbeit, 3,* 25–29.

Matern, U., & Waller, P. (1999). Instruments for minimally invasive surgery: Principles of ergonomic handles. *Surgical Endoscopy, 13,* 174–182.

Matern, U., Waller, P., Giebmeyer, C., Rückauer, K. D., & Farthmann, E.H. (2001). Ergonomics: Requirements for adjusting the height of laparoscopic operating tables. *Journal of the Society of Laparoendoscopic Surgeons, 5,* 7–12.

7 Anesthesia Incidents and Accidents

Matthew B. Weinger
University of California, San Diego
Veterans Administration San Diego Healthcare System

ANESTHESIOLOGIST, WILLIAM JONES, M.D.

Dr. William Jones completed his anesthesiology residency training only last year. The 3 years of training were grueling—long hours, little time off, challenging clinical cases taking care of really sick people. His marriage did not survive the experience. Bill was now looking forward to going into private practice, to finally be able to make some money and have time to relax and enjoy life. He had no idea that private practice would not be much different from his residency.

Bill joined a group of anesthesiologists in St. Louis. Because he was the new guy, he seemed to get all of the worst work shifts—nights, weekends, and holidays. He worked like a dog and was constantly exhausted. Although his paychecks were a huge increase over a resident's salary, Bill was surprised to find how little was left at the end of each month after paying for his malpractice insurance, living expenses, student loans, and alimony to his ex-wife.

About 6 months after he joined, Bill's group was awarded a contract to provide anesthesia services at Fulgom Hospital and Bill was assigned to work there. The hospital was busy; they did all kinds of surgery, usually until late in the evening. In addition, because Fulgom Hospital was the regional trauma center, one of the anesthesiologists had to stay in the hospital all night in case there was an emergency surgery.

The operating rooms at Fulgom Hospital were new and well equipped. Bill was not that familiar with their new Nioda anesthesia workstations because where he had trained they used older Gratel anesthesia machines. The 500-pound Nioda, with all of its fancy electronic displays and computer options, struck Bill as unnecessarily complicated. Fortunately, for routine cases, Bill could ignore most of the Nioda's extra features.

Bill remembers vividly his first night on call. In his nearly 5 years of anesthesia training and practice, it was the first time a patient had died under his care. It was only his first week and he was still trying to get oriented. In addition, he was fighting off a cold and had been tempted to call in sick, but decided not to because he was new and the group already was short-handed.

Starting at 7 a.m., Bill worked all day doing routine outpatient cases. It was a good thing that the antihistamine/decongestant pills kept his nose from running or he would have been miserable wearing a soaking wet sterile mask on his face all day. Bill had a quick dinner, and then as emergency cases stacked up — an appendectomy, a broken leg, a bleeding stomach ulcer — he continued to work despite increasing fatigue and sleepiness as well as discomfort from his ever-worsening cold. After 11 p.m., he was the only anesthesiologist in the hospital.

At 3:30 a.m., Bill finally was able to lie down. He could not have been dozing for more than a few minutes when his beeper sounded. He was being called emergently to Operating Room (OR) #8, the one designated for trauma cases. Stumbling out of bed and rubbing sleep out of his eyes, Bill ran to OR #8 where he first met Belinda Jefferson, who was already lying on the electronic operating room bed. It was cold in the OR and Bill shivered as he began to assess the situation. There were six nurses and surgeons huddled around Mrs. Jefferson, busy removing her clothes and preparing her for surgery. The white ceramic tile walls reflected the bright light and made the sound of people talking, the clanging of surgical instruments, and the ever-present radio music seem even louder than usual.

Mrs. Jefferson was a 38-year-old woman who appeared to weigh about 300 pounds. Bill was told by the trauma surgeon that Mrs. Jefferson got in a fight in a bar and was shot three times with a handgun; in her right chest, right upper abdomen, and left thigh. Mrs. Jefferson did not look good — she was pale and writhing in pain. Bill attached the routine anesthesia monitors to her. They confirmed what he suspected: her blood pressure was very low (80/40), and her heart rate of 120 beats per minute was fast. These readings were consistent with her having already lost a lot of blood. In addition, her injured lungs were not very effectively saturating her blood with oxygen. Bill tried to ask Mrs. Jefferson if she had any other medical problems but she was largely incoherent; her diminished mental capacity could have been due to her low blood pressure, the inadequate oxygen supply to her brain, or the effects of the alcohol Bill could smell on her labored breath.

The surgeons were eager to begin their work quickly to rescue Mrs. Jefferson. Bill started to prepare his anesthesia supplies, drugs, and equipment. He needed to anesthetize Mrs. Jefferson and place a special upside-down Y-shaped breath-

ing tube into her windpipe. This breathing tube not only would allow him to keep her anesthetized with anesthesia gases, it also would separate her lungs so the surgeons could work on the injured right lung while Bill continued to ventilate the left one. Because of her critical condition, Bill attached additional monitors. He placed a plastic catheter in the artery in her wrist to monitor her blood pressure with each beat of her heart. After she was asleep, he also planned to insert a longer plastic catheter through the skin of her neck into her jugular vein and down into her heart to allow monitoring of how much blood was getting back to her heart and how effectively the heart was beating.

It took Bill more time than he would have liked to get prepared because he was still unfamiliar with how the anesthesia supply cart was organized. It did not help that the head surgeon, Dr. Hartzel, was yelling at him to hurry up and anesthetize Mrs. Jefferson so he could start operating; he had never before worked with Dr. Hartzel. Bill had to open every drawer of the cart before he found all of the dozens of things he needed. Finally he was ready. Bill took a deep breath, and then asked Mrs. Jefferson to do the same through the oxygen mask she was wearing. He administered a small dose of an anesthesia drug into the intravenous line that went right into Mrs. Jefferson's blood stream. As she suddenly became still and quiet, it did not dawn on Bill that she would never again regain consciousness.

ISSUES

The story about Bill and Mrs. Jefferson, which continues in segments throughout this chapter, is fictitious; however, nearly every aspect of it occurs regularly. With the narrative as a platform, this chapter provides a picture of the anesthesiologist's job and some of the error-related factors that impact contemporary anesthesia care   factors that affected Dr. Bill Jones as he anesthetized and cared for Mrs. Jefferson.

The Effects of Fatigue on Anesthesiologist Performance

Bill Jones was fatigued due to overwork and acute sleep loss.

Anesthesia residents, individuals who, after completing 4 years of medical school and a 1-year internship, are pursuing further training in the medical specialty of anesthesiology, work an average of 73 hours per week including night and weekend responsibilities (Howard, Healzer, & Gaba, 1997). Some work weeks may exceed 100 hours. Many fully trained practicing physicians similarly work extended hours. When on call, anesthesiologists typically work 24-hour shifts, often without sleep. Unlike many other medical specialties, anesthesiology has fostered a culture that discourages providing clinical care after a night on call in which there was acute sleep loss. In spite of this, private practice anesthesiologists often provide care for a short list of identified routine surgical cases the morning after they have worked the preceding day and night. Even a single night of sleep loss, as when on call, produces appreciable fatigue and sleepiness, a depressed mood, and reduced motivation to perform that could lead to an adverse incident (Weinger & Ancoli-Israel, 2002).

An extended work week, encompassing long, challenging shifts and inadequate restorative sleep—conditions that are common for anesthesia residents—leads to chronic fatigue. Indeed, many anesthesia residents are chronically sleep deprived. Despite not having been on call for at least 2 full days, anesthesia residents placed in a dark room during the middle of the day of a regular work week, fell asleep as quickly as would individuals with narcolepsy (Howard, Gaba, Rosekind, & Zarcone, 2002). Acute or chronic lack of sleep impacts cognitive processes that are critical for safe anesthesia care. Sleep-deprived physicians may have impaired learning and thought processes, memory deficits, irritability, and interpersonal dysfunction as well as degraded job performance (Weinger & Englund, 1990). Fatigued individuals pay less attention to peripherally located instruments and are inconsistent in their response to external stimuli. When coping with task demands, fatigued persons exhibit less control over their own behavior and tend to select more risky alternatives or short cuts.

People who work excessively long hours not only experience sleep deprivation, they also are affected by the disruption of their normal circadian rhythm (their sleep–wake cycle), which leads to further fatigue and performance impairment. In most sustained work activities, major decrements usually occur after 4 hours and again after 18 hours (Alluisi & Morgan, 1982). Performance decrements may actually appear more rapidly when monitoring or vigilance tasks, such as those required of the anesthesiologist, are involved. The magnitude of performance impairment after remaining awake for 24 hours is roughly equivalent to being legally drunk (Dawson & Reid, 1997).

Efforts by state legislatures and licensing bodies to regulate residents' clinical work schedules have generally met with resistance. This is due primarily to cultural constraints—the long work hours are considered a rite of passage for new physicians—and, more importantly, the economic realities of physician staffing in underfunded, understaffed urban academic medical centers where a majority of residents train.

Ambient Conditions in the Operating Room

Bill's work environment is cold and noisy.

Temperature.   Uncomfortable environmental temperatures, a common situation in many ORs, can impair performance (Ramsey, 1983). People tend to exhibit unsafe behaviors that could lead to occupational injury when temperatures fall outside a preferred range of 17°C to 23°C. Thus, temperatures in the OR, which can be as low as 7°C in some adult ORs or approach 30°C in ORs for pediatric or burn patients, could lead to unsafe behaviors and adverse outcomes.

Noise. It has been said that "the noise level in the OR frequently exceeds that of a freeway" (Shapiro & Berland, 1972). Typical ambient noise in the modern OR ranges from a level equivalent to the sound of a vacuum cleaner (at about 70 decibels) to that of a nearby accelerating motorcycle (about 90 decibels). Because of the need for sterility and ease of cleaning, the walls, floor, and ceiling of the OR usually are covered with a material such as ceramic tile, which not only precludes significant noise damping, but also reflects every sound back into the room. High noise levels are produced by the various pieces of equipment such as the patient ventilator (that breathes for the anesthetized patient) and the vacuum system that suctions surgical fluids or blood from the wound (up to 96 decibels). Conversations among the OR personnel and sometimes loud background music further contribute to the cacophony.

High levels of noise such as in the OR detrimentally affect short-term memory (Hockey, 1978) and may also mask task-related cues or cause distractions during critical activities (Poulton, 1978), as well as interfere with effective verbal communication. In addition, loud noise has the potential to impair decision-making during critical events (Weinger & Englund, 1990).

State of Health

Bill was working despite having a cold and taking therapeutic medications.

Physicians, like the patients they care for, develop illnesses. However, the medical culture and work pressures make it difficult for physicians to admit illness or even fatigue. Anesthesiologists experience significant pressure to avoid case cancellations, minimize the time between cases, to not complain, and to work when ill, fatigued, or otherwise not at their best (Gaba, Howard, & Jump, 1994). Succumbing to these pressures and working when one's abilities may be compromised can predispose to unsafe conditions, as may the cognitive effects of medications taken for the illness. Many commonly prescribed medications, including some antihistamines, antidepressants, cough suppressants, and pain relievers, have measurable effects on mental functioning and alertness.

Interpersonal and Team Factors

Bill had never before worked with Dr. Hartzel, who was now yelling at him.

Team communication is critical and involves unspoken expectations, traditions, general assumptions regarding task distribution, chain-of-command hierarchies, and individual emotional and behavioral components. Alterations in any of these factors can impair effective team function (Kanki, Lozito, & Foushee, 1989). Ineffective communication between health care providers has been shown to contribute to the occurrence of clinical errors (Donchin et al., 1995). The anesthesiologist must function as an integral part of the OR team. Many personal interactions in the OR can affect the anesthesiologist's perform-ance adversely, for example, dealing with a difficult surgeon or an uncooperative nurse. In highly complex tasks involving teamwork, the team performs best if it has been together for a long time and is well practiced. In critical situations, team members must make a special effort to communicate clearly and unam-biguously. Yet, it is under stressful conditions when individual and team per-formance is most likely to deteriorate. Communication may prove even more difficult when some or all of the team members are fatigued or under stress.

Bill took over Mrs. Jefferson's breathing by holding a rubber mask tightly over her mouth and nose with his left hand while rhythmically squeezing a rubber bag pressurized with oxygen with his right hand to fill her lungs with each emp-tying of the breathing bag (see Fig. 7.1). Bill then administered a paralytic drug to make it even easier to breathe for Mrs. Jefferson during the surgery. He watched the monitor display as Mrs. Jefferson's blood pressure dropped still further from the toxic effects of the anesthesia medication on her heart. No one has yet discovered a drug that reliably produces loss of consciousness without undesirable side effects like reduction of the contractile strength of the heart, or dilation of the blood vessels leading to pooling of the blood in the legs and reduced blood flow back to the heart.

Fortunately, Bill was able to counteract the low blood pressure with the injec-tion of an adrenaline-like drug that makes the heart beat faster and stronger. A minute later, once Mrs. Jefferson's lungs were full of oxygen, Bill inserted a long lighted metal tongue blade (called a laryngoscope) into her mouth and, apply-ing steady upward and outward traction, was able to visualize her vocal cords. He quickly placed the breathing tube through her vocal cords and down into her two main bronchi (windpipes) so that the right and left sides of the double lumen breathing tube ventilated the right and left lungs independently.

A nurse began to scrub most of Mrs. Jefferson's exposed body with brown iodine soap as Bill performed a variety of other necessary tasks. He inserted a long tube through Mrs. Jefferson's nose into her stomach and placed a ther-mometer into her esophagus. Bill lubricated and taped shut her eyes so they would not be accidentally scratched during what he expected to be a long and involved surgery. Then, as the surgeon made a deep scalpel incision into Mrs. Jefferson's abdomen, Bill became engrossed in the insertion of the plastic moni-toring catheter through her neck and into her heart.

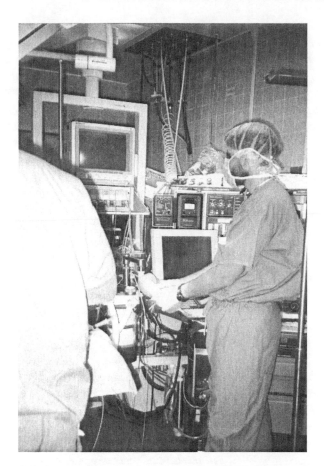

FIG. 7.1.   An anesthesiologist squeezes the "breathing bag" attached via tubing to a patient's lungs (not shown) to breathe for the anesthetized patient. The anesthesiologist simultaneously observes the patient's blood pressure, heart rate, and other vital signs. The multiple controls and displays of the complex anesthesia workstation are partially seen behind the physician.

Things proceeded as well as one could expect, at least for the next hour. As the surgeons worked on Mrs. Jefferson's abdominal injuries, Bill needed to replace the intravenous fluids and blood she lost. Occasionally, Mrs. Jefferson's blood pressure would decrease when the surgeons lost too much blood too quickly. At these times, Bill had to turn off the anesthesia drugs because they could lower the blood pressure even further. When he had time, Bill tried to maintain a detailed written record of everything he did for Mrs. Jefferson. Bill was exhausted and he knew he was not functioning at his best; it took all of his concentration to focus on the most immediate tasks at hand. Thus, Bill failed to notice the earliest signs of trouble.

Mrs. Jefferson was developing malignant hyperthermia (the second word meaning increased temperature), a rare genetic disease that most commonly manifests itself first under anesthesia. In malignant hyperthermia (or MH), some anesthesia drugs trigger a sudden increase in the amount of calcium inside the skeletal muscle cells, leading to excessive activation of the body's metabolism. Because of Mrs. Jefferson's other medical problems, Bill did not even think of MH when her heart rate increased; he attributed it to surgical bleeding and the necessarily light anesthetic state.

Bill was so busy coping with other things, he did not notice the increased amounts of carbon dioxide in the gas Mrs. Jefferson exhaled from her lungs, an early sign of tissue acidosis. Unfortunately, the auditory alarms of the Nioda anesthesia machine had never been turned on, precluding an early notification of the higher-than-normal levels of carbon dioxide in the breathing tubing of the machine. Unbeknownst to Bill, the hospital's biomedical engineering department had, in response to complaints from the nurses about auditory alarms sounding repeatedly in empty operating rooms, decided to reconfigure the Nioda's internal software so that when it was first turned on, the auditory alarms were disabled.

Bill failed to notice the only indication that the auditory alarm system was disabled, a small red symbol of a bell with an X through it in the upper left corner of the primary data display. If the alarms had been activated, Bill would have heard an auditory warning to direct his attention to the elevated exhaled carbon dioxide and also Mrs. Jefferson's increased body temperature. It was only when Mrs. Jefferson's heart began to beat irregularly (due to the high levels of acid in her blood) that Bill put all the clues together and realized that his patient was in serious trouble.

Anesthesia Devices

Bill was unfamiliar with the anesthesia machine he was using and did not recognize that the auditory alarms were disabled.

Anesthesiologists tend to use medical devices in the same way they use automobiles; they expect that a new device will work more or less the same as equivalent older devices (Mosenkis, 1994). Bill knew that the new anesthesia machine at Fulgom Hospital had a number of features that the older machine he trained on did not. However, Bill, like most other anesthesiologists, believed that what he already knew about the older machine would be applicable to the newer one. His experience did not prepare him to look for a relatively subtle indication that the alarms were disabled. It would have been much better for Bill, and for Mrs.

Jefferson, if the new machine's design allowed it to be operated correctly without training or even consulting the manual (Mosenkis, 1994).

As is often the case, although on first glance this incident might be attributed solely to human error, it was, in fact, exacerbated by the design of the anesthesia machine, which effectively hid the indication that the alarms were disabled. Although the percentage of anesthesia mishaps that are primarily due to equipment failure appears to be relatively small (Cooper, Newbower, Long, & McPeek, 1978), the contribution to error of suboptimal equipment design, maintenance, implementation, or performance may be significant. Designers of anesthesia equipment have attempted to aid the anesthesiologist by incorporating devices to augment vigilance and enhance clinical performance. Alarms, intended to notify the operator of potentially critical situations, are only effective if properly designed and implemented.

Vigilance and Anesthesiology Job Performance

Bill failed to detect several early cues of the impending crisis.

Vigilance is a state of readiness to detect and respond to specific small changes occurring at random intervals in what is observed (Mackworth, 1957). In anesthesia, the need for vigilance may be most apparent during the quiescent period of the maintenance phase of a routine anesthetic—the time during surgery that begins after the induction (or initiation) of the anesthesia state and ends as the patient starts to emerge from anesthesia. During maintenance, the anesthesiologist must continuously monitor and evaluate the patient's medical status while assessing the effects of anesthesia and surgical intervention. This involves higher order cognitive processes such as pattern recognition, the ability to divide attention among and to prioritize multiple tasks, and the ability to make decisions under time pressure and the stress of incipient patient injury (Gaba, Howard, & Small, 1995).

A number of factors can adversely affect clinical vigilance such as inexperience or inadequate supervision, increased stress, task complexity, or faulty equipment design (Weinger & Englund, 1990). The number and type of tasks required, as well as the speed of their performance vary throughout each anesthetic (Gaba & Lee, 1990; Weinger et al., 1994). As clinical conditions demand greater attention during more complex aspects of an anesthetic or during a critical event, the anesthesiologist transitions from a low-workload, monitoring-oriented, task scenario to a more cognitively demanding active response scenario. Under high workload conditions, secondary tasks are neglected, anesthetic routine may be disrupted, and attention focused on those demanding conditions may reduce vigilance for lower priority or uncommon clinical cues (Loeb, 1994; Weinger, Herndon, & Gaba, 1997; Weinger et al., 1994).

Once Bill appreciated all of the clinical cues, especially given that Mrs. Jefferson's body temperature was now 102°F, he immediately made the diagnosis of malignant hyperthermia (MH). Although he had never before seen a case, the topic had been discussed many times in his residency training and so he knew basically what to do. He immediately turned off all of the anesthesia agents, delivered 100% oxygen to Mrs. Jefferson, and told the surgeons that a crisis was developing. The operating room was suddenly quiet. Dr. Hartzel asked Bill what they should do. Bill began to bark out orders. He told the nurses to bring in buckets of ice to cool Mrs. Jefferson and to call the pharmacy to immediately bring a quantity of dantrolene, the specific treatment for an MH crisis, to OR #8. The sooner Mrs. Jefferson received the drug, the better her prognosis.

Unfortunately, there was a 20-minute delay before the dantrolene arrived. No patient at Fulgom Hospital had ever experienced an MH crisis, and there was no established protocol. The pharmacist on call was new; he had to call a supervisor at home to find out where they kept the drug. Neither Bill nor anyone in the OR had ever mixed dantrolene; it took them more than an hour to dilute and administer the more than 100 vials that Mrs. Jefferson's body size required. Bill had immediately called the back-up anesthesiologist, Dr. Rugerb, but by the time she arrived to help, Mrs. Jefferson's condition was irreversible; she never regained consciousness. She died 2 days later from failure of most of her major body organs because their cells had been damaged by the acidosis and high temperature. The hospital ordered an inquiry into the appropriateness of Dr. Jones' clinical care. A few months later, Mrs. Jefferson's family filed a medical malpractice suit against the hospital and Dr. Jones.

On-the-Job Stress

Bill suddenly found himself in a new and highly stressful situation.

Sources of stress affecting job performance come from the work environment itself, which includes both social and physical stressors (Raymond, 1988), the tasks involved such as mental workload and pacing of activity, and the characteristics of the individual involved including health, fitness, and personality. Factors in the individual's life, such as financial worries or a recent fight with a spouse, can adversely impact job performance and even increase the likelihood of accidents (Bignell & Fortune, 1984).

The extent to which stress, such as what Bill experienced in caring for Mrs. Jefferson, affects a person is evidenced by physiological changes that are analogous to those that prepare the body to fight or flee from a threat. One's heart rate, blood pressure, and respiratory rate all increase. Although rarely considered, what a person eats and drinks can contribute to stress. Caffeine is considered by many to enhance mental performance; however, even among regular coffee drinkers, caffeine ingestion can magnify the physiological consequences of stress (Lane & Williams, 1987).

Emergency procedures are more stressful because of the critical importance of a timely response to the situation. Anesthetic emergencies, such as malignant hyperthermia, produce a greater physiological stress response in clinicians than do routine anesthetics, and this effect is more profound in less experienced clinicians. Even during a routine procedure, such as placing a breathing tube into the patient's windpipe, novice anesthesia residents exhibit a greater stress response than do more experienced anesthesia providers (Loeb, Weinger, & Englund, 1993; Weinger et al., 1994). Training and experience reduce the stress and workload associated with emergency situations, which points to the value of formal Crisis Resource Management training (Gaba, Fish, & Howard, 1994).

The Role of Human Error in Anesthesia Mishaps

It is important to emphasize that serious adverse events are relatively uncommon in anesthesia and, when they occur, it is often difficult retrospectively to separate the human from system factors (Leape et al., 1995; Runciman, Webb, Lee, & Holland, 1993). Many adverse clinical events appear to be the result of multiple system factors such as reimbursement policies, workload, or the design of equipment over which individual clinicians have little control (Bogner, 1994; Donchin et al., 1995; Leape et al., 1995; Runciman, Webb, et al., 1993). However, the anesthesia provider has traditionally been considered a contributor to the occurrence of most anesthesia mishaps (Gaba, 1989; Gaba & DeAnda, 1989; Keenan & Boyan, 1985; Weinger & Englund, 1990; Williamson, Webb, Sellen, Runciman, & Van der Walt, 1993). In fact, before the importance of system factors was widely appreciated, clinician errors were said to account for up to 75% of anesthetic mishaps (Cooper et al., 1978; Keenan & Boyan, 1985). Readers who would like more detailed information on human error in anesthesia are referred to several additional sources (Arnstein, 1997; Gaba, 1989; Runciman, Sellen, et al., 1993; Weinger & Englund, 1990).

Common sense suggests that inexperienced clinicians make more mistakes, leading to lower quality patient care. Indeed, a relationship exists between clinical experience, represented by the number of procedures performed, and patient outcomes (Houghton, 1994; Konrad, Schupfer, Wietlisbach, & Gerber, 1998; Rosser, Rosser, & Savalgi, 1997; See, Cooper, & Fisher, 1993). Anesthesiologists with greater, more varied experience are generally able to respond to untoward events more effectively than less well trained clinicians (Gaba & DeAnda, 1989; Kurrick, Devitt, & Cohen, 1998).

Experienced anesthesia providers are able to perform more clinical tasks per minute and are more efficient in their actions than are novice anesthesia residents

(Weinger et al., 1994). The experienced clinicians also report working less hard and are able to detect a visual alarm more quickly than novices. These differences are likely to be greater during complex or critical clinical situations. It is important to emphasize that clinical experience can be viewed as a systems factor in that well-established educational, licensing, credentialing, and staffing policies determine the amount of training and experience each individual clinician attains throughout his or her career. Similarly, the assignment of inexperienced clinicians to difficult cases without adequate supervision or back-up is a systems issue.

System Factors Play a Critical Role in the Occurrence of Anesthesia Mishaps

During a 6-month period in one hospital, a diabetic patient's left leg was mistakenly amputated instead of his right leg, a ventilator-dependent patient in the ICU died because the wrong patient was allowed to breathe on his own, and a patient under anesthesia for a cesarean section was mistakenly subjected to a post-partum tubal ligation. The official explanation for all three of these incidents was that personnel failed to follow established verification procedures; however, a detailed evaluation of such incidents inevitably reveals a chain of events involving multiple factors beyond those of the individuals involved in the incident (Gaba, 1989; Weinger & Englund, 1990).

Errors can stem from many factors including conditions that impair effective communication, difficult-to-use devices, operational policies or procedures that conflict with actual operational requirements, pressures to perform more efficiently or cost-effectively, or inadequate quality control over clinical processes. Good operating practice is essential but may not be sufficient to prevent errors. The likelihood of an adverse event may be determined not by the anesthesiologist's skill in caring for the patient but by factors such as fatigue from working long hours or a device that is so complex that it facilitates use errors. The anesthesiologist's personal condition as well as the condition of his or her equipment and the OR environment needs to be optimal to assure the most successful response to a difficult or critical clinical situation.

On the surface, Mrs. Jefferson might appear to be the only victim of this unfortunate scenario. Yet, Dr. Bill Jones, a dedicated, motivated, and competent anesthesiologist, also was a victim. Many factors contributed to Mrs. Jefferson's unfortunate demise; however, a negligent anesthesiologist was not one of them. Mrs. Jefferson arrived in the operating room that night in a compromised state; her obesity, inebriation, and injuries reduced her body's recuperative reserve and placed her at risk for a bad outcome when her dormant malignant hyper-

thermia was triggered by the anesthesia. Bill also was in a compromised state: He was fatigued, sleep deprived, not feeling well because of the cold he was catching, and possibly affected by the medication he took for his cold. Perhaps he should have refused to work under these circumstances; however, by doing so he certainly would have upset his colleagues and possibly lost his job.

Being relatively new to the practice and the hospital, Bill was unfamiliar with the nuances of his equipment and his work environment. Despite excellent clinical training, he had never before actually managed a malignant hyperthermia crisis. The hospital did not have adequate procedures for maintaining equipment, communicating with clinicians about new or altered equipment, or for managing malignant hyperthermia. Although all of these issues came out in Mrs. Jefferson's family's lawsuit, the attorneys for both Fulgom Hospital and the insurance company that had the policy for Bill's anesthesia group elected to settle out of court. The settlement against Dr. Jones was reported to the National Practitioner Data Bank and to the State Medical Board.

The allegations and recriminations took a heavy toll on Bill; he left the anesthesia group and Fulgom Hospital soon thereafter. Bill Jones relocated to another city and continued to practice anesthesiology for many years. Similar stories have ended in compounded tragedy: a vicious cycle of guilt, substance abuse, and ultimately even death—tragedies that might have been prevented by addressing the systems factors that contribute to error.

ACKNOWLEDGMENTS

Preparation of this chapter was possible thanks to the support of the Agency for Healthcare Research and Quality (AHRQ P20-HS11521 and R01-HS11375, Rockville, MD) and the Veterans Administration's Health Services Research and Development Service (IIR 20–066, Washington, DC). Over the years, many students, research assistants, colleagues, and collaborators contributed to our research and my understanding of the issues covered in this chapter.

REFERENCES

Alluisi, E. A., & Morgan, B. B. (1982). Temporal factors in human performance and productivity. In E. Alluisi & E. E. Fleishman (Eds.), *Human performance and productivity. 3: Stress and performance effectiveness* (pp. 165–247). Hillsdale, NJ: Lawrence Erlbaum Associates.
Arnstein, F. (1997). Catalogue of human error. *British Journal of Anaesthesia, 79,* 645–656.
Bignell, V., & Fortune, J. (1984). *Understanding system failures.* Manchester, England: Manchester University Press.
Bogner, M. S. (1994). *Human error in medicine.* Hillsdale, NJ: Lawrence Erlbaum Associates.

Cooper, J. B., Newbower, R. S., Long, C. D., & McPeek, B. (1978). Preventable anesthesia mishaps: A study of human factors. *Anesthesiology, 49,* 399–406.

Dawson, D., & Reid, K. (1997). Fatigue, alcohol and performance impairment. *Nature, 388,* 235.

Donchin, Y., Gopher, D., Olin, M., Badihi, Y., Biesky, M., Sprung, C., Pizov, R., & Cotev, S. (1995). A look into the nature and causes of human errors in the intensive care unit. *Critical Care Medicine, 23,* 294–300.

Gaba, D. (1989). Human error in anesthetic mishaps. *Internal Anesthesia Clinics, 27,* 137–147.

Gaba, D., & DeAnda, A. (1989). The response of anesthesia trainees to simulated critical incidents. *Anesthesia and Analgesia, 68,* 444–451.

Gaba, D. M., Fish, K. J., & Howard, S. K. (1994). *Crisis management in anesthesiology.* New York: Churchill Livingstone.

Gaba, D. M., Howard, S. K., & Jump, B. (1994). Production pressure in the work environment. California anesthesiologists' attitudes and experiences. *Anesthesiology, 81,* 488–500.

Gaba, D. M., Howard, S. K., & Small, S. D. (1995). Situation awareness in anesthesiology. *Human Factors, 37,* 20–31.

Gaba, D. M., & Lee, T. (1990). Measuring the workload of the anesthesiologist. *Anesthesia and Analgesia, 71,* 354–361.

Hockey, G. R. J. (1978). Effects of noise on human work efficiency. In D. E. May (Ed.), *Handbook of noise assessment* (pp. 335–372). New York: Van Nostrand Reinhold.

Houghton, A. (1994). Variation in outcome of surgical procedures. *British Journal of Surgery, 81,* 653–660.

Howard, S. K., Gaba, D. M, Rosekind, M. R., & Zarcone, V. P. (2002). The risks and implications of excessive daytime sleepiness in resident physicians. *Academic Medicine, 77*(10), 1019–1025.

Howard, S. K., Healzer, J. M., & Gaba, D. M. (1997). Sleep and work schedules of anesthesia residents: A national survey [abstract]. *Anesthesiology, 87,* A932.

Kanki, B. G., Lozito, S., & Foushee, H. C. (1989). Communication indices of crew coordination. *Aviation, Space, and Environmental Medicine, 60,* 56–60.

Keenan, R. L., & Boyan, P. (1985). Cardiac arrest due to anesthesia. *Journal of the American Medical Association, 253,* 2373–2377.

Konrad, C., Schupfer, G., Wietlisbach, M., & Gerber, H. (1998). Learning manual skills in anesthesiology: Is there a recommended number of cases for anesthetic procedures? *Anesthesia and Analgesia, 86,* 635–639.

Kurrick, M. M., Devitt, J. H., & Cohen, M. (1998). Cardiac arrest in the OR: How are our ACLS skills? *Canadian Journal of Anaesthesia, 45,* 130–132.

Lane, J. D., & Williams, R. B. (1987). Cardiovascular effects of caffeine and stress in regular coffee drinkers. *Psychopharmacology, 24,* 157–164.

Leape, L. L., Bates, D. W., Cullen, D. J., Cooper, J., Demonaco, H. J., Gallivan, T., Hallisey, R., Ives, J., Laird, N., Laffel, G., Nemeskal, R. Petersen, L. A., Porter, K., Servi, D., Shea, B. F., Small, S. D., Sweitzer, B. J., Thompson, B. T., & Vander Vliet, M. (1995). Systems analysis of adverse drug events. *Journal of the American Medical Association, 274,* 35–43.

Loeb, R., Weinger, M. B., & Englund, C. E. (1993). Ergonomics of the anesthesia workspace. In J. Ehrenwerth & J. B. Eisenkraft (Eds.), *Anesthesia equipment: Principles and applications* (pp. 385–404.). Malvern, PA: Mosby Year Book.

Loeb, R. G. (1994). Monitor surveillance and vigilance of anesthesia residents. *Anesthesiology, 80,* 527–533.

Mackworth, N. H. (1957). Some factors affecting vigilance. *Advancement of Science, 53,* 389–393.

Mosenkis, R. (1994). Human factors in design. In C. W. D. van Gruting (Ed.), *Medical devices* (pp. 41–51). Amsterdam, The Netherlands: Elsevier.

Poulton, E. (1978). A new look at the effects of noise: A rejoinder. *Psychological Bulletin, 85,* 1068–1079.

Ramsey, J. (1983). Heat and cold. In G. Hockey (Ed.), *Stress and fatigue in human performance* (pp. 33–60). Chichester, England: John Wiley and Sons.

Raymond, C. (1988). Mental stress: "Occupational injury" of 80's that even pilots can't rise above. *Journal of the American Medical Association, 259,* 3097–3098.

Rosser, J. C., Rosser, L. E., & Savalgi, R. S. (1997). Skill acquisition and assessment for laparoscopic surgery. *Archives of Surgery, 132,* 200–204.

Runciman, W. B., Sellen, A., Webb, R. K., Williamson, J. A., Currie, M., Morgan, C., & Russell, W. J. (1993). Errors, incidents, and accidents in anaesthetic practice. *Anaesthesia and Intensive Care, 21,* 506–519.

Runciman, W. B., Webb, R. K., Lee, R., & Holland, R. (1993). System failure: An analysis of 2000 incident reports. *Anaesthesia and Intensive Care, 21,* 684–695.

See, W. A., Cooper, C. S., & Fisher, R. J. (1993). Predictors of laparoscopic complications after formal training in laparoscopic surgery. *Journal of the American Medical Association, 270,* 2689–2692.

Shapiro, R., & Berland, T. (1972). Noise in the operating room. *New England Journal of Medicine, 287,* 1236–1238.

Weinger, M., & Englund, C. (1990). Ergonomic and human factors affecting anesthetic vigilance and monitoring performance in the operating room environment. *Anesthesiology, 73,* 995–1021.

Weinger, M. B., & Ancoli-Israel, S. (2002). Sleep deprivation and clinical performance. *Journal of the American Medical Association, 287,* 955–957.

Weinger, M. B., Herndon, O. W., & Gaba, D. M. (1997). The effect of electronic record keeping and transesophageal echocardiography on task distribution, workload, and vigilance during cardiac anesthesia. *Anesthesiology, 87,* 144–155.

Weinger, M. B., Herndon, O. W., Paulus, M. P., Gaba, D., Zornow, M. H., & Dallen, L. D. (1994). Objective task analysis and workload assessment of anesthesia providers. *Anesthesiology, 80,* 77–92.

Williamson, J. A., Webb, R. K., Sellen, A., Runciman, W. B., & Van der Walt, J. H. (1993). Human failure: An analysis of 2000 incident reports. *Anaesthesia and Intensive Care, 21,* 678–683.

8 The Trojan Horse of the Operating Room: Alarms and the Noise of Anesthesia

F. Jacob Seagull
University of Maryland

Penelope M. Sanderson
The University of Queensland, Australia

ANESTHESIOLOGIST, DR. JESSICA PINDAR

Dr. Jessica Pindar is a 33-year old M.D. anesthesiologist who has been practicing for 6 years in public hospitals. She now works at Burnham Memorial Hospital—a large public hospital in the inner Chicago area. Burnham Memorial has an extensive operating suite that exposes her to a wide variety of cases. Working at Burnham Memorial also exposes Jessica to quite a range of anesthesia equipment. Different components of Burnham Memorial's operating suite have different equipment, some of which was purchased at different times in the past and still is in use; other specific types of equipment were purchased to meet the needs of the different specialties. Senior anesthesiology consultants in a given specialty, such as cardiac surgery, learn about new equipment from colleagues, conference presentations, and sales representatives, then they press Burnham Memorial's administrators to buy new equipment in their specialty. Quite often, rather than order the doctors' preferred make and model of a piece of equipment, the administrators substitute a more cost-effective make and model.

The equipment Jessica uses in the operating room (OR) includes an anesthesia machine that delivers anesthetic gas to patients to put them to sleep; the patient monitoring system that displays patients' vital signs so she can check that the patients are safe; and infusion pumps (computer-chip-based devices) that deliver intravenous drugs at programmed rates of flow to the patient as needed throughout surgery. Anesthesia technicians, who traditionally are trained to work with the mechanical aspects of the anesthesia equipment but have no medical or nursing certification, set up the anesthesia machine before Jessica arrives in the OR. Each piece of equipment has its unique quirks in functioning that anesthesia care providers (ACPs), including Jessica, get to know as they use it. If equipment malfunctions or if quirks require workarounds (ways of compensating for problems) that are unsafe, the ACPs can send equipment to the biomedical engineering department where specialist engineers and technicians fix it, as their workload and level of training allows.

It is the end of Mr. Fitzpatrick's surgery and he still is unconscious. As one of her responsibilities, Jessica must move her patients from the operating table to a wheeled gurney and transport them from the OR to the recovery room at the end of the corridor, where they will wake up or emerge from the anesthetic under the care of recovery room nurses. Jessica has finished disconnecting Mr. Fitzpatrick from the regular monitors in the OR and OR personnel have connected him to several pieces of portable equipment for the trip to the recovery room. This process usually involves managing a spaghetti-like array of wires from various medical devices including the electrocardiograph (ECG) that monitors the activity of the heart and the pulse oximetry system that monitors the concentration of oxygen in the blood, as well as several intravenous lines that carry drugs into Mr. Fitzpatrick's veins from portable infusion pumps.

During the transition from OR to portable equipment, Mr. Fitzpatrick receives high-flow 100% oxygen delivered through a face mask from a rather large oxygen tank in a wire holder at the foot of the bed. Also loaded onto the foot of Mr. Fitzpatrick's bed are his medical chart, all the paperwork from the surgery he has just undergone, and the small transport monitor that displays his ECG, oxygen saturation, and other vital signs. The continuous beep sound of pulse oximetry was turned off because Mr. Fitzpatrick's oxygen saturation could be read from the display on the transport monitor.

Jessica walks at the foot of the bed as Mr. Fitzpatrick is wheeled from the OR to the recovery room so she is near enough to the transport monitor to read the rather dim, small LCD digital display if needed. The transport monitor suddenly emits a high-pitched beep. The particular transport monitors that Burnham Memorial bought a year ago were the least expensive of the options considered. Unfortunately, those monitors have the reputation of being erratic; that is, alarms sound often, usually either because of a loose connection or because a slight movement of the patient creates an artifact signal that triggers the alarm. "It's those cheap transports again," grumbles the anesthesia technician at the head of the bed. From long habit, Jessica presses the Silence Alarms button on the transport monitor to stop the sound. Because false alarms are commonplace and thought to be meaningless, she does not take the time to bend down to read the LCD display.

Further down the corridor they turn into the recovery room where waiting recovery room nurses and technicians help guide Mr. Fitzpatrick's bed into its bay. Three people are disconnecting Mr. Fitzpatrick from the transport equipment and connecting him to the patient monitoring system on the wall of the recovery room, as well as switching his oxygen supply from the tank to the wall unit. During this time, Jessica picks up the chart and anesthesia record from the foot of Mr. Fitzpatrick's bed and turns to the recovery nurse to give a report of his progress under anesthesia and how he currently is doing.

Mr. Fitzpatrick now is properly connected to the recovery room monitoring system and no alarms are sounding. Jessica sees that whatever caused the transport monitor to alarm apparently had reflected problems with the transport monitor, rather than any danger to the patient, who is now stirring slightly at the start of another safe emergence from anesthesia at Burnham Memorial Hospital.

THE WORLD OF THE ANESTHESIA CARE PROVIDER

To understand Jessica's world and the role equipment alarms play in it, we first must understand what an ACP does in and around the OR. The ACP has responsibility for patients from the time they are taken from the preoperative area and brought into surgery until after completion of surgery when they are handed over to qualified recovery room personnel. The ACP uses gases and intravenous drugs to induce a state of anesthesia in the patient and assumes responsibility for maintaining all the vital physiological functions that anesthesia suppresses. The ACP must monitor the patient's level of consciousness as well as his or her cardiovascular signs such as heart rate, blood pressure, and the blood oxygen level.

For those types of anesthesia that inhibit the patient's ability to breathe spontaneously, ACPs control the ventilation (breathing) of the patient by either manually squeezing a bag attached to a face mask to push air into the patient's lungs (referred to as bagging) or with a mechanical ventilator attached to the mask, which uses motor-driven mechanical bellows to accomplish the same task. The patient also may be intubated by placing a tube into the patient's trachea that leads to the lungs and attaching the tube to the bag or to the ventilator. To be certain the patient is properly ventilated, the ACP monitors the measurements of various parameters associated with breathing such as respiration rate, inspired (inhaled) oxygen level, expired (exhaled) carbon dioxide level (capnography), airway pressures, and tidal (breath) volume. (See Baskett, Dow, Nolan, & Maull, 1994, for well-illustrated descriptions of anesthesia and critical care procedures and equipment.)

During surgery, the ACP usually works at the patient's head with an anesthesia machine, similar to the one shown in Fig. 8.1, which provides anesthetic gases and agents, the ventilator, and additional patient monitoring systems, all of which are stacked above the anesthesia machine and comprise one side of the care provider's workspace. On the other side of the ACP, seen in the foreground of Fig. 8.1, is a cart that contains drugs and other supplies. Quite often because of constraints of the physical environment, the anesthesia machine and monitor-

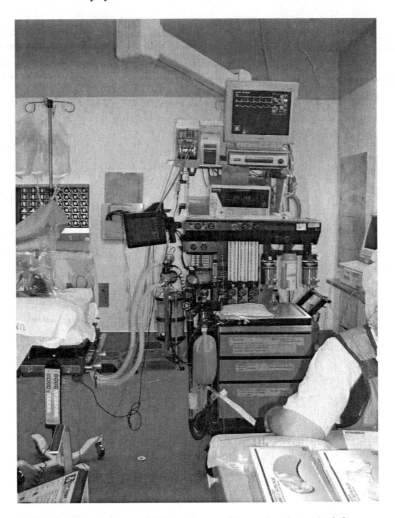

FIG. 8.1.   A typical anesthesia workspace. The patient is on the left, connected to the anesthesia machines and other patient-monitoring systems, seen centrally, and the supply cart, seen in the foreground, is across from the anesthesia machine.

ing systems are behind the ACP as he or she faces the patient, which appears to be the case in Fig. 8.1. The surgical team works on the patient's body unless the operation involves the head, as in brain surgery. Sterile drapes typically separate the patient's head, the domain of the ACP, from the rest of the patient's body, the domain of the surgical team. The drapes often obscure the ACP's view of the surgery.

While the patient is in the operating room, the ACP determines what the normal range is for the patient's vital signs from the patient's medical chart, and tracks deviations from that range. The ACP determines if the deviations are spontaneous, drug-induced, or surgery-induced. In addition, the ACP notes in the anesthesia record (a legal requirement) the drugs delivered, interventions performed, and patient vital signs throughout surgery.

Connecting the patient to the anesthesia machine and the monitoring devices at the beginning of each operation and disconnecting them at the end often causes alarms to sound when there actually are no problems. Technology cannot distinguish whether a patient has been disconnected purposefully, accidentally, or whether a major change occurred in the monitored function. Contextual factors are used by ACPs to distinguish meaningful changes from a normal state of affairs. Sometimes a low heart rate is very worrisome and requires medication. At other times—for example, just after anesthesia is induced and before surgery starts—low heart rates are expected and are tolerated because the start of surgery will increase a low heart rate even when a person is anesthetized. Furthermore, because no two patients are the same, there is uncertainty as to what constitutes normal and abnormal states.

Jessica continually is interacting with alarms: She uses alarms in a variety of ways to help meet the multiple demands on her as well as determining the meaning of the sounding alarms. Jessica's experiences with the alarms as the day progresses—including the ways she uses them to help her as she performs anesthesia on her list of patients who come into the OR for surgery one after the other—is illustrated by the next patient on her list, Mr. Kramer, a 58-year-old man in for routine knee surgery.

Jessica knows from Mr. Kramer's preoperative assessment that he is a non-smoker, has no known allergies, and generally is in good health. She greets Mr. Kramer as he is wheeled in the OR, lying on the gurney. After connecting him to the electrocardiogram, the pulse oximeter, and infusion pumps, Jessica delivers the drugs that induce anesthesia. Because it is expected to be a short case, Jessica has induced a light anesthesia that nonetheless suppresses Mr. Kramer's breathing. Rather than attaching Mr. Kramer to a mechanical ventilator, Jessica elects to keep his lungs working manually by bagging him through his face mask. Members of the surgical team are preparing to start when Jessica suddenly hears a continuous beep of a nearby alarm. After a moment or two, everyone looks up from his or her activities; the continuous sound indicates that corrective action probably has to take place before the alarm will stop.

"It's the battery alarm from the infusion pump," states an anesthesia technician approaching the pump to deal with it, but that is not the problem. Jessica looks at the display screen of the patient monitor for an indication of an unusual variation in Mr. Kramer's vital signs; she sees none. The surgeon frowns and calls out, "Is someone doing something about that ventilator alarm?" Jessica finds no alarm coming from the ventilator. It is difficult to determine which device is alarming because all the alarms in the OR sound quite similar. While she continues to bag Mr. Kramer, Jessica directs the anesthesia technician to check each piece of equipment for an alarm or an indication of a problem that would cause an alarm. No alarms are found from any of the obvious pieces of equipment. The alarm does not seem to be coming from any particular direction, which is puzzling. Jessica turns her head to do a quick visual check of Mr. Kramer and the alarm seems louder.

"Do operating tables now have alarms too?" Jessica jokes. She and the anesthesia technician start peering around the table while she continues to bag Mr. Kramer. It takes them a few minutes to determine that the alarm sound comes from the hearing aid that inadvertently was not removed from Mr. Kramer's ear during preoperative preparation. When his head was moved slightly as bagging began, the hearing aid started to feed back a high-pitched beep that sounded like one of the many alarms heard each day in the OR. The hearing aid is removed and the "alarm" sound stops.

Jessica's experience underscores how the alarms in the OR are indistinguishable. Even the people who constantly hear OR alarms cannot discriminate among them or identify a new sound. Anesthetists almost invariably find it necessary to examine their displays and equipment to determine what an alarm means. Spending time searching for the source of an alarm delays fixing the underlying cause, which could have serious consequences when the problem is a significant change in patient status.

Surgery begins. Jessica must record the drugs and the quantities of them she used to induce anesthesia for the anesthesia record. She also must record Mr. Kramer's vital signs every 5 minutes. Until now she has been squeezing the ventilator bag with her preferred left hand, but she needs to use her left hand for writing. The anesthesia machine's work area, however, is designed for right-handed ACPs who write with their right hand while bagging the patient with their left. Jessica has learned to accommodate to this by crossing her arms in front of her body as illustrated in Fig. 8.2, so her right hand is squeezing the ven-

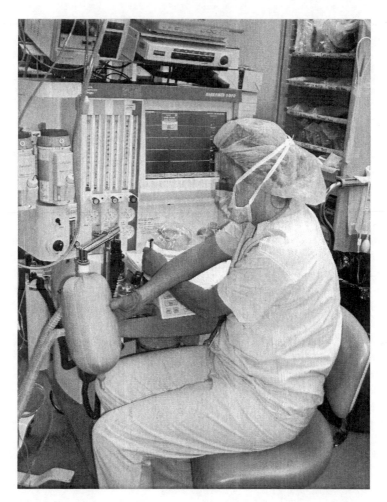

FIG. 8.2. An awkward position for a left-handed person. Anesthesia machines typically provide writing space that is convenient only for right-handed people. To write and "bag" simultaneously requires this awkward crossed-arm position.

tilator bag on her left. That way she can use her preferred left hand to write in the anesthesia record in front of her. To write legibly, Jessica pauses in squeezing the ventilator bag and uses her right hand to keep the paper from sliding while she writes on it. If she does this for too long, the ventilator beeps to indicate that no breathing is detected, which reminds her to start squeezing the ventilator bag again. Although this is awkward, it is the best she can do to get everything completed on time given the brevity of the surgical procedure, the necessity of charting the anesthesia record, and working in an OR designed for right-handed ACPs—all at the same time.

After about 10 minutes, when she is not charting in the record, Jessica is joined by Ivan, a new anesthesia resident who has started working with her. They begin talking about the recently implemented cost-cutting measures at Burnham Memorial. Jessica is interested in the discussion and squeezes the bag a little less frequently. The ventilator alarm sounds again. As Jessica turns to squeeze the bag, she does not notice that just at the same time, Ivan hits the switch to silence the monitor alarms. She turns back to the discussion with Ivan. After about 15 seconds Jessica realizes she has not squeezed the ventilator bag and as she does so as she realizes that the ventilator alarm did not sound to remind her, as it had before. She quickly checks the capnography and oximetry monitors to determine if the respiration and oxygenation of the blood are normal and finds the effect of the extended pause in ventilation clearly evident. To determine why the alarm did not sound, Jessica looks at the monitor and sees the indication that the alarms have been silenced for 2 minutes.

"Did you silence the alarms just then, Ivan?" she asks. When he says yes, she explains that she was using the ventilator alarm to remind her to keep bagging while charting or doing other tasks. "That was dangerous," she says. "The alarm is my reminder to ventilate Mr. Kramer. If I don't ventilate him, his oxygen saturation will decrease and his heart rate will increase, but I wouldn't know that for a long time if the alarms are silenced."

Jessica was alert and recognized what happened before it led to problems. Like many ACPs, when pressed for time she uses the alarm for a purpose beyond that originally intended. She uses the fact that the machine registers a failure to ventilate by an alarm as a reminder to her to ventilate. The time pressure of the series of short surgeries on her list, the need to chart throughout surgery, and the layout of her workspace that is unsympathetic to her left-handedness have led her to exploit the alarm. Using the alarm as a reminder is creative, but as she recognizes, it has its vulnerabilities. Later in the same case, however, Jessica will use the ability to silence the alarms in the same creative way that she used the active alarms.

As the case progresses, the surgeon realizes that Mr. Kramer's condition requires more extensive surgery than anticipated, necessitating a longer time in surgery and deeper anesthesia. Near the end of the surgery, Mr. Kramer's heart rate becomes a little high and the heart rate alarm sounds by giving a loud beep. The alarm will repeat the loud beep every 30 seconds until Mr. Kramer's heart rate returns to normal. At the sound of the alarm, the surgeon looks up with a questioning look; she is notorious for wanting a quiet operating theatre. Jessica is looking at the monitor to determine what is causing the alarm. Mr. Kramer's heart rate is 92 beats per minute. This is higher than the normal rate of around 70 beats per minute, but not so high as to necessitate treating it with drugs, especially with the surgery nearing its end. The alarm sounded because Jessica set the warning for the upper limit heart rate at 90; 92 is above 90. Jessica could set the upper heart limit to 100 so the alarm will not sound again unless Mr. Kramer's heart rate continues to climb until it is over 100. Jessica is wary of doing that: anything above 90 is really too high and she wants to know about it. She wants to keep close track of the vital signs even if it involves hearing the alarm from time to time. She also wants to know when Mr. Kramer's heart rate falls below 90. If she keeps the upper limit at 90, she will know when this happens because the alarm will stop sounding. If she sets the upper limit to 100, however, no heart rate below 100 will set off the alarm.

As Jessica considers her options, the heart rate alarm goes off again. To reduce the noise in the OR, hence avoid the wrath of the surgeon, Jessica silences the alarm. Because the alarm silence button silences all alarms on the monitor, no alarm will sound for the next 2 minutes for any variation in any vital sign sensed by the monitor. If Mr. Kramer's heart rate is still above the upper limit of 90 when the 2-minute silence period is over, the alarm will sound and Jessica will probably reduce the noise level by silencing the alarms again. On the other hand, if the 2-minute period of silencing ends and Mr. Kramer's heart rate is below 90, no alarm will sound. Jessica knows that if this occurs while her attention is drawn elsewhere, she might not notice the lack of alarm. However, she believes this is a safe practice because if no alarm starts to sound when the alarm-silencing period ends, then Mr. Kramer's heart must have returned to the normal range.

Despite the fact that ACPs such as Jessica need to know one of three things about the patient's heart rate—if it is the same, has drifted up to a level that requires treatment, or has returned to normal—the monitoring equipment is not designed to give this information. Like many ACPs, Jessica approximates this kind of information by using the heart rate alarm limit as a baseline, and continuing to silence the alarm. Obtaining information this way comes at the cost of quite a bit of work. Moreover, if the heart rate suddenly goes up while the alarms are silenced and Jessica has not been watching the visual information on the monitor, an important event might be missed. Even worse, if something quite different happens, such as a drop in blood pressure or a rise in temperature, Jessica will not be alerted to that until the next time she visually scans the monitor. Jessica's efforts to compensate for the monitor not providing needed information will work when the patient's condition essentially is steady, and when there are no unexpected occurrences.

Late that day, Jessica is tired from being on her feet administering anesthesia for over 8 hours. Mr. Blevsky's surgery, the second from the last on Jessica's afternoon list, takes longer than expected because the surgeon needs to control bleeding prior to final suturing. Eventually the surgical team finishes and leaves the OR to clean up, take a short break, and prepare for the delayed final surgery of the day. "Let's get the last patient on the list prepped as soon as possible," says the surgeon as she leaves. Jessica remains because she must transport Mr. Blevsky to the recovery room and hand him over to the recovery staff. Mr. Blevsky is still unconscious. Jessica and Ivan finish disconnecting him from the monitors in the OR, transfer him from the operating room table to the gurney, and connect him to several pieces of portable equipment for the trip to the recovery room. "Ivan," says Jessica, "could you please bring our final patient in here and get him prepped while I transport Mr. Blevsky to recovery?"

At this point, Mr. Blevsky is breathing on his own, and is on high-flow oxygen through a face mask. Resting on the foot of Mr. Blevsky's bed is the same assortment of items as for Mr. Fitzpatrick at the start of the day, including the small transport monitor that displays vital sign readings. The anesthesia technician helps Jessica and an OR nurse guide the bed toward the recovery room. Typically, as with Mr. Fitzpatrick, Jessica walks at the foot of the bed, glancing over the documents she is about to pass on to the recovery room nurse. The transport monitor soon lets out a high-pitched beep. "Not again," grumbles the anesthesia technician. Jessica has a fleeting recollection of the transport alarm with Mr. Fitzpatrick earlier in the day. "I don't think I've had a single transport this week without a pointless alarm," she comments. Jessica presses the Silence Alarms button on the transport monitor to stop the sound; she does not investigate further.

When they turn into the recovery room, Mr. Blevsky's space is not ready. It is still occupied by 66 year-old Mrs. Carbone who, as she was being moved to a general ward to provide space for Mr. Blevsky, suddenly complained of strong chest pains. Recovery room personnel have gathered; they are concerned that Mrs. Carbone will have a heart attack, as she has a history of them. Some personnel are reattaching her ECG wires so they can monitor the activity of her heart. Others are pulling a special crash cart toward her bed in anticipation of needing to administer drugs and defibrillate her heart to normalize its beat should she experience cardiac arrest. There is no place for Mr. Blevsky's bed; however, Mrs. Carbone is in good hands. As the person with the most senior medical qualifications on the scene, Jessica will be expected to take a leadership role if Mrs. Carbone goes into cardiac arrest. Jessica knows that the recovery room personnel have noted that she is nearby and she experiences a small anticipatory rush of adrenaline. Mr. Blevsky's transport monitor alarms again and she quickly silences it while assessing the entire situation.

If Mrs. Carbone cannot leave recovery, then there is no recovery bay for Mr. Blevsky, so he will have to remain on the transport monitor under qualified care until a bay is available. Alternatively, Jessica could take him back to the induction area in the OR; however, they know that Ivan is transporting the next patient for surgery to their OR. Nothing can be worked out for Mr. Blevsky until the situation with Mrs. Carbone is resolved; Jessica must remain nearby. The anesthesia technician returns to the OR to investigate their options. "Watch him for a moment," Jessica says to the OR nurse who has transported Mr. Blevsky with her. She walks over to Mrs. Carbone's bed. Mrs. Carbone is pale now with clammy skin, and looks up at Jessica in pain but also in trust. As Jessica examines the ECG and oxygen saturation signals on the monitor above her bed, Mrs. Carbone's heart rhythm deteriorates rapidly into cardiac arrest. The scene erupts with activity and multiple monitor alarms sound as the protocol for handling a cardiac arrest unfolds. Neither Jessica nor the OR nurse with Mr. Blevsky hears the transport monitor sound its alarm again. Jessica coordinates the protocol for a well-practiced, life-saving scenario for Mrs. Carbone, calling for the administration of appropriate drugs, CPR, chest compressions, and attempts to shock the heart back into a healthy rhythm with the defibrillator. Additional medical personnel arrive quickly as the crisis is announced in coded form over the hospital public address system; soon Mrs. Carbone's heart beat returns to normal and her eyes open. "You gave us a bit of a fright just then, Mrs. Carbone, but you're OK now," says Jessica kindly. She turns to an anesthesiologist colleague who has come to the scene and says, "Jim could you please take charge? I'm transporting a patient right now."

The OR nurse has been keeping Mr. Blevsky physically protected from the rush of activity while trying to determine if he can be returned to the OR area. As Jessica approaches, she sees that the OR nurse has just discovered a serious deterioration in Mr. Blevsky's condition indicated by his oxygen saturation reading and bluish skin tone. "Jessica, his sats (saturation levels) have dropped through the floor and he's cyanotic (blue)," she says in an alarmed voice. Jessica touches Mr. Blevsky's skin and twists around quickly and peers down so she can read the transport monitor's display properly. She sees the classic readouts for hypoxia, lack of oxygen. Mr. Blevsky's face mask was to be giving him high-flow 100% oxygen from the tank. Jessica quickly checks whether the oxygen is flowing and finds it is not. The tank was not properly connected to the oxygen line and Mr. Blevsky has been breathing room air all this time.

The 21% oxygen concentration of room air was not adequate for Mr. Blevsky at this point in his recovery from anesthesia. The transport monitor had an alarm to indicate the problem, but every time the alarm sounded Jessica assumed it was a quirk and silenced it. If the pulse oximetry sound had been on, the drop in oxygen saturation would have been indicated aurally. If the LCD panel had been easier to read, it might have been consulted more regularly and the pulse oximetry value seen. Jessica and the OR nurse had been in a dilemma with Mr. Blevsky—they were unable to take him to a recovery bay and probably unable to take him back to the OR. The alarms caused by Mrs. Carbone's cardiac arrest drowned out the alarm from the Mr. Blevsky's transport monitor, and the possibility of an imminent life-threatening situation drew Jessica as the senior medical professional to Mrs. Carbone's side.

Later tests revealed that Mr. Blevsky probably had experienced some brain damage from the hypoxia sustained during his transport. He sued, and the next year was a professional nightmare for all involved at Burnham Memorial.

ISSUES

Alarms are widely acknowledged to be a problem in critical care environments: They do not give useful information when it is needed and often are intrusive (Cook & Woods, 1996; Seagull & Sanderson, 2001). Every incident or activity Jessica encountered is typical of what occurs. There is a great deal of irony with alarms: They were introduced in the early 20th century at the instigation of medical insurance companies, but because of their poor fit with the nature of the critical care work and environment within which they function, they sometimes contribute to adverse outcomes rather than prevent them (Hyman & Drinker, 1983; Weinger, 1995). The following discussion addresses systems factors that can make alarms hazardous rather than helpful.

Origin of False Alarms

In the typical operating room, an alarm sounds every 4.5 minutes; 75% of them are false alarms (Kestin, Miller, & Lockhart, 1988). An alarm can be a false alarm either because it reflects an artifact of measurement such as from the sensor being jostled, static electricity, or from oversensitivity, or because it provides the ACP unimportant or already known information. False alarms are an endemic problem; if they happen frequently, ACPs become desensitized to them and are less likely to pay attention to them and respond appropriately (Kestin, Miller, & Lockhart, 1988; Meredith & Edworthy, 1995; Xiao, Mackenzie, Jaberi, Harper, & the LOTAS Group, 1996). In other words, false alarms have a cry-wolf effect (Breznitz, 1984) in that people tend not to respond to an alarm they consider false even if the alarm indeed is valid (Bliss, Gilson, & Deaton, 1995).

The cry-wolf effect was evident at the beginning and end of Jessica's day when the transport monitor alarm sounded but was silenced without further investigation. From her experience, Jessica discounted the alarm with Mr. Fitzpatrick, the first patient in the story, thinking it had been electronic noise created by the movement of the bed, which is a quirk of an inexpensive machine. It also could have been a loose ECG wire, which is such a commonplace occurrence that a recovery room nurse would probably not bother noting it when reconnecting Mr. Fitzpatrick to the recovery room equipment. Alternatively, it could have been a lack of oxygen flow from the cylinder, just as it was for Mr. Blevsky. Jessica did not determine which of these possibilities was the cause of the alarm. Evidently, from his physical appearance, Mr. Fitzpatrick never was in danger. Despite the alarms, the fact that the patient clearly was healthy reinforced the belief that the transport monitor was quirky and produced uninformative and unimportant alarms, which reduced the likelihood that alarms would be investigated rather than simply silenced.

Beliefs that alarms are false lead ACPs to silence them. Sixty-eight percent of a group of Canadian ACPs deactivated an alarm at some point at the start of a case because they anticipated too many false alarms; 12% deactivated an alarm at the start of a case because the alarms were uninformative due to auditory confusion with sounds in the OR (McIntyre, 1985).

Audibility, Discriminability, and Identifiability of Alarm Sounds

The incident with Mr. Kramer's hearing aid illustrates a basic issue—namely, how difficult care providers find it to recognize the source of a given alarm. Jessica and her colleagues could not determine that the sound of the hearing aid was not an alarm. In addition, the alarms from the various patient sensors for a given monitor tend to sound the same and often are distinguished only by the severity of the alarm, with minor problems being signaled by a single alarm chime or beep and more severe problems signaled by a series of two or three chimes. In Mr. Kramer's case, when his heart rate started to increase, Jessica had to look at the monitor display to determine the specific problem; the alarm indicated only that a problem existed.

ACPs find it difficult to reliably identify what a given alarm within many alarms in the OR indicates—they are accurate only about 50% of the time (Block, 1988; Cropp & Woods, 1994; Loeb, Jones, Leonard, & Behrman, 1992). Indeed, patient deaths have been attributed to confusions about which piece of equipment was alarming (Meredith & Edworthy, 1995). The louder and more urgent-sounding alarms are responded to more quickly regardless of the under-

lying importance of the problem (Meredith & Edworthy, 1995; Xiao, Mackenzie, et al., 1996).

Hidden within the various sounds in an OR and other technology-intensive
settings such as an Intensive Care Unit (ICU), important alarms may go unheard.
This happened when Jessica was attending to Mrs. Carbone's cardiac arrest in
the recovery room and a cacophony of monitor alarms from that situation was
sounding. Neither Jessica nor the OR nurse heard the additional alarm from the
transport monitor at the end of Mr. Blevsky's bed. The number of alarms that
sound can be overwhelming for ACPs. Only a few of the alarms are signaling the
actual cause of the problem, whereas others are signaling redundant information
(Mackenzie, Martin, Xiao, & the LOTAS Group, 1996), and some alarms are not
detected simply because of masking by ambient noise (Momtahan, Hetu, &
Tansley, 1993).

Hybrid Equipment with Hybrid Alarms

In the OR and other critical care environments, equipment tends to consist of
piecemeal collections rather than an integrated suite of monitoring and control
devices. This was the case at Burnham Memorial; Jessica had to use assorted
medical devices that had been purchased for specialized purposes at different
times. In addition, she often had to search for a piece of equipment because the
placement of the devices varied in the larger ORs used for cardiac and other prolonged surgery compared to the smaller rooms for some of the shorter procedures, and was different still from the critical care settings. Integrating information such as the numerous vital signs into a single source may allow intelligent
filtering and elimination of nuisance alarms (Blom, 1988; Loeb, Brunner, Westenskow, Feldman, & Pace, 1989; Mylrea, Orr, & Westenskow, 1993; Navabi,
Mylrea, & Watt, 1989; Orr & Westenskow, 1994). Without such integration, the
ACPs must perform the integration and mental filtering themselves, often when
there are additional cognitive demands due to changes in the patient's condition.

Alarms as Tools for Unsupported Work Contexts

Alarms originally were developed to alert ACPs to a measure that had deviated
beyond an acceptable range. This design is based on the assumptions that the
ACP would be regularly checking the patient's vital signs, and also that the same
numerical deviation would always have the same meaning for the ACP (Xiao &
Seagull, 1999). In contrast to the intended use, Jessica used the alarms as
reminders to ventilate the patient while responding to the competing demands of
creating the patient's anesthesia record. ACPs use alarms for reasons other than
having their attention directed to variations in physiological measures that might

otherwise go unheeded (Seagull & Sanderson, 2001; Stanton, 1994; Woods, 1995), as illustrated by Jessica using the alarm to monitor variations in Mr. Kramer's heart rate. Using integrated monitors that filter out many of the alarms would limit the ACPs' ability to use the alarms creatively to cope with unforeseen demands in their work (Xiao & Seagull, 1999).

Competing Noise

Noise is endemic in critical care environments (Hay & Oken, 1972) and is a leading cause for burnout in ICU staff (Topf & Dillon, 1988). Alarms are at the top of the list of noise sources.

Surgical procedures can last for hours and be tedious; care providers differ in how they handle the tedium. The surgeon and the physician-anesthesiologist are, in principle, professional equals and colleagues. Because the activities of surgeons are the most apparent, they very often assume the positions of leadership and presume their preferences will prevail. During Mr. Kramer's case, Jessica worked with a surgeon who was well known for wanting a quiet OR—in other words, as few alarms interrupting the quiet as possible so that everyone can focus on his or her tasks. Jessica weighed the options for configuring the monitoring of her patient so as few alarms as possible would be emitted yet be consistent with patient safety. Indeed, in the Canadian study of alarm use (McIntyre, 1985), the need for peace and quiet was the reason 26% of the ACPs deactivated an alarm system at some point during the start of a case. Other surgeons, however, are less concerned about the sound of alarms and may want music playing during some phases of the surgery or encourage a conversational atmosphere in the OR to enhance the working environment. All sounds in the setting compete with alarms for auditory attention.

Physical Environment

Jessica's left-handedness illustrates an obvious yet unresolved issue with the physical layout of the anesthesia work area: the OR typically is organized for right-handed people. While charting against time pressure, Jessica relied on the ventilator alarm to alert her to the need to ventilate the patient if for some reason she paused in doing so. The composition of the physical environment did not support the task to be done to such an extent that Jessica had difficulty meeting the minimal demands of patient ventilation.

The physical layout of the anesthesia workspace in general leaves much to be desired, and the arrangements of equipment have been described as haphazard at best (Drui, Behm, & Martin, 1973; Harper, Jaberi, Mackenzie, & LOTAS, 1996; Kennedy, Fiengold, Wiener, & Hosek, 1976; Weinger & Englund, 1990).

The placement of equipment with the usual viewing angle of 130° to 170° between the patient and monitoring equipment makes it nearly impossible for the ACP to see the patient and the patient's vital signs simultaneously (McIntyre, 1982).

Team Factors

Anesthesia care providers are members of a team that includes nurses, surgeons, technicians, and others who provide care for the patient during surgery. The composition of such teams changes with every case, and even within the span of a single case. ACPs are affected by the changing team composition, changing responsibilities, and the dynamics of multiple actors in the medical environment. (For a comprehensive review of issues in team performance in the operating room, see Helmreich & Schaefer, 1994.) Jessica discussed work-related issues with Ivan, the new resident, during her case with Mr. Kramer. Later, when Mrs. Carbone had a heart attack in the recovery room, Jessica became the head of an ad hoc emergency resuscitation team. Each of these changes compromised Jessica's ability to hear and respond appropriately to alarms.

In his attempt to help Jessica manage the alarms by silencing them for her, Ivan inadvertently foiled her use of the alarms as a reminder. It is common for staff nearby to silence alarms, if they believe the primary ACP noticed the alarm but was engaged in other tasks. Because of the lack of communication between Ivan and Jessica, Ivan's effort for efficient teamwork actually threatened patient safety.

On arriving at the recovery room and recognizing the dilemma of having no space for Mr. Blevsky, Jessica and the team that transferred him to the recovery room had to redefine their roles. Direct responsibility for Mr. Blevsky was in transition, passing between teams, when the situation was compounded by the alarms from Mrs. Carbone's monitors masking the transport monitor alarm. Such unexpected events strain the care-provider team's ability to cope with the complexity of providing care. Indeed, team coordination has not been effective in team responses to emergency cases (Ben-Barak et al., 1999; Xiao, Hunter, et al., 1996; Xiao, Mackenzie, Patey, & the LOTAS Group, 1998), to the extent that team coordination and communication failures have been cited as contributing to adverse patient outcomes in two of every three hospitals (Joint Commission on Accreditation of Healthcare Organizations, 2000).

Alarms affect teamwork because different ACPs use monitors in each OR differently, and those uses typically are not coordinated across the ACPs. At the beginning of the day when the patient monitor is turned on, the default alarms that have been set for the specific OR or critical care unit are activated. As each patient with a different physiological condition is connected to the monitor, the alarm limits may be increased or decreased as appropriate. When ACPs change, as when an ACP relieves another during a long case, the new ACP must be aware of the alarm limits; otherwise, alarms may be misinterpreted. This points to the importance of communication and coordination not only with those providing different aspects of care, but also among those providing the same type of care.

Organizational, Legal, and Economic Factors

Jessica and her medical colleagues were under pressure to finish cases quickly so Burnham Memorial could meet the demand for its services in the most timely and cost-effective way. This is typical of trends in health care in the late 1990s and early 2000s. Each successive surgical case is started sooner after the end of the previous case than in less cost-conscious times. Because of this, administrative and other nonsurgical tasks must be completed during surgery. In addition, patients are anesthetized as lightly as possible for a short recovery time, which means less time in the recovery room and faster discharge for same-day surgery. Light anesthesia, however, requires increased ACP vigilance to ensure that anesthesia is adequate for the patient to be free of pain.

Despite the need for vigilance, the anesthesia record must be kept current because it is a legal document that the hospital must retain. In addition to the anesthesia record, Jessica had the task of using the bag to ventilate the patient and had other competing demands with little time to meet them because the cases were relatively short. Using the alarm as a reminder to keep ventilating the patient while she complied with regulations and maintained the anesthesia record was an adaptive response to a highly pressured situation.

As the result of cost cutting imposed by reimbursement policies, there are fewer staff physicians and qualified nurses in hospitals than before such constraints were imposed. This was evident for Jessica when she interacted with anesthesia technicians who often are not as knowledgeable nor are they paid as much as registered nurses. Because of reduced staffing, when arriving at the recovery room with Mr. Blevsky, Jessica was the only physician present when Mrs. Carbone experienced the cardiac arrest. That crisis diverted Jessica's attention from the issue of whether the transport monitor alarms were false or valid alarms.

ADVERSE OUTCOMES REFLECT SYSTEMS ISSUES

Jessica's experiences highlight the fact that adverse outcomes are the result of multiple system factors that impact the care provider, rather than the result of an

act perpetrated solely by an individual. It is always possible to point to a super-
ficial reason for an accident but it is impossible to find a single underlying cause
(Senders & Moray, 1991). In other words, Mr. Blevsky's hypoxia and his subsequent brain damage can be explained in terms of the events that led to those conditions and so provide a reason the accident happened, but it is much more difficult to determine the underlying causes of those events and why the precursor
events occurred (Bogner, 1994, 2000). This is particularly so when the focus is
only on the individual associated with the incident. When the context of care
is analyzed from the perspective of the involved individual, however, incident-
provoking factors within the system as a whole can be identified and altered to
prevent such an incident from happening again.

Incidents have been discussed in terms of the combination of circumstances
that led to them: the busy OR list, the full-to-capacity recovery room, the low-
cost monitor with its occult alarms considered false alarms, the acoustic masking effect of multiple alarms in a crowded environment, the cramped workspace
for the ACP, the teamwork protocols reorienting priorities when emergencies
occur, and the concern with keeping Mr. Blevsky out of physical harm from the
activity surrounding the cardiac arrest.

Although the typical response to an incident with an adverse outcome is to
attribute it to human error, that response does not answer the question of why the
error occurred. In Mr. Blevsky's case, assume for the sake of discussion that the
full recovery room was the fault of the scheduler of the busy OR. The question
must be asked—Why? The response most likely would be that due to fiscal constraints, each surgery is allotted a certain amount of time for completion and the
hours available for surgery must be filled to be cost effective. Thus, the busy OR
was not the fault of the scheduler, but of the systems factor of the reimbursement
policies that mandated the tight scheduling of the OR.

Similarly, purchase of the low-cost transport monitors that emit an inordinate
number of false positive alarms typically would be attributed to the chair of the
hospital committee that decided to purchase them. The response to why that
decision was made might identify the committee's belief that a hospital policy
exists to purchase the lowest cost product and the extant hospital policy to accept
that committee's recommendation without question. Once identified, the belief
and the policy can be reviewed for their impact on patient safety and subsequently modified to avoid inappropriate purchases in the future.

Despite considering systems factors, the typical target for attributing the
cause of an adverse outcome is the care provider associated with the incident.
The ultimate question is the culpability of the care provider. Given the time pressure of the OR list and the quirks of her equipment, Jessica might have avoided
Mr. Blevsky's outcome had she checked every setting on every device every
time it was used and investigated every alarm even though the vast majority of

alarms were uninformative, but that would have slowed the hospital's work and possibly jeopardized Mr. Blevsky's outcome by prolonging his surgery, as well as jeopardizing the outcomes of the patients whose surgery was delayed. Health care providers want to and typically do perform to the highest standards, yet the conditions in which they must work and the situations in which they find themselves are comprised of error-provoking system factors that accumulate and lead to adverse outcomes.

The snapshot of the work of an anesthesiologist, Jessica Pindar, illustrates the multiple ways health care providers accommodate the awkward characteristics of alarms and the events that precipitate them. The strategies that Jessica employed throughout the day are all an accepted part of normal anesthesia practice. As her conversation with Ivan indicated, Jessica was a vigilant ACP, educated in the possibility of error arising from the way alarm systems are used, and actively involved in communicating that possibility to a trainee. Such errors might be interpreted as the result of the workarounds Jessica used; however, the actual causes were the system factors that made workarounds necessary, such as the design of the physical environment for right-handed people. Therefore, rather than presume that adverse outcomes originate in human error, an understanding of why an error occurs can be achieved from analyzing the context in which the incident occurred to determine the system factors that contribute to the adverse outcome. Only through this systems approach can errors be meaningfully interpreted.

REFERENCES

Baskett, P. J. F., Dow, A., Nolan, J., & Maull, K. (1994). *Practical procedures in anesthesia and critical care.* London: Mosby.

Ben-Barak, S., Inselbuch, M., Hyams, G., Straucher, Z., Michaelson, M., Gopher, D., Tal-Or, E., & Klein, Y. (1999, June 15–17). Teamwork in a complex system: An analysis of a hospital shock-trauma unit. *Proceedings of the International Conference on TQM and Human Factors—toward successful integration.* Linkoping, Sweden.

Bliss, J. P., Gilson, R. D., & Deaton, J. E. (1995). Human probability matching behavior in response to alarms of varying reliability. *Ergonomics, 38,* 2300–2313.

Block, F. E. (1988). Evaluation of users' abilities to recognize musical alarm tones. *Journal of Clinical Monitoring, 8,* 285.

Blom, J. A. (1988). Real-time expert systems in patient monitoring. *Journal of Clinical Monitoring, 4,* 130–131.

Bogner, M. S. (1994). *Human error in medicine.* Hillsdale, NJ: Lawrence Erlbaum Associates.

Bogner, M. S. (2000, November 20–24). Stretching the search for the "why" of error: The systems approach. *Proceedings of the Fifth Australian Aviation Psychology Symposium.* Manly, Australia.

Breznitz, S. (1984). *Cry wolf: The psychology of false alarms.* Hillsdale, NJ: Lawrence Erlbaum Associates.

Cook, R. I., & Woods, D. D. (1996). Adapting to new technology in the operating room. *Human Factors, 38,* 593–613.

Cropp, A. J., & Woods, L. A. (1994). Name that tone: The proliferation of alarms in the intensive care unit. *Chest, 105*(4), 1217–1220.

Drui, A. B., Behm, R. J., & Martin, W. E. (1973). Predesign investigation of the anesthesia operational environment. *Anesthesia and Analgesia, 52,* 584–91.

Harper, B. D., Jaberi, M., Mackenzie, C. F., & LOTAS. (1996). Increasing efficiency in the Trauma Resuscitation Anesthesia workspace. *Anesthesiology, 85*(3A) [Abstract], A378.

Hay, D., & Oken, D. (1972). The psychological stresses of intensive care nursing. *Psychosomatic Medicine, 34,* 109–118.

Helmreich, R. L., & Schaefer, H. (1994). Team performance in the operating room. In M. S. Bogner (Ed.), *Human error in medicine* (pp. 225–253). Hillsdale, NJ: Lawrence Erlbaum Associates.

Hyman, W. A., & Drinker, P. A. (1983). Design of medical device alarm systems. *Medical Instrumentation, 17,* 103–106.

Joint Commission on Accreditation of Healthcare Organizations (2000, February 4). Operative and post-operative complications: Lessons for the future. *Sentinel Event Alert, 12.* Available online: http://www.jcaho.org/about+us/news+letters/sentinel+event+alert/print/sea_12.htm

Kennedy, P. J., Fiengold, F., Weiner, E. L., & Hosek, R. S. (1976). Analysis of task and human factors in anesthesia for coronary artery bypass. *Anesthesia and Analgesia, 55,* 374–377.

Kestin, I. G., Miller, B. T., & Lockhart, C. H. (1988). Auditory alarms during anesthesia monitoring. *Anesthesiology, 69,* 106.

Loeb, G. J., Brunner, J. X., Westenskow, D. R., Feldman, B., & Pace, N. L. (1989). The Utah anesthesia workstation. *Anesthesiology, 70,* 999–1007.

Loeb, R. G., Jones, B. R., Leonard, R. A., & Behrman, K. (1992). Recognition accuracy of current operating room alarms. *Anesthesia and Analgesia, 74,* 499–505.

Mackenzie, C. F., Martin, P., Xiao, Y., & the LOTAS Group (1996). Video analysis of prolonged uncorrected esophageal intubation. *Anesthesiology, 84*(6), 1394–1403.

McIntyre, J. W. R. (1982). Man–machine interface: The position of the anesthetic machine in the operating room. *Canadian Anesthesia Society Journal, 29,* 74–78.

McIntyre, J. W. R. (1985). Ergonomics: Anaesthetists' use of auditory alarms in the operating room. *International Journal of Clinical Monitoring and Computing, 2,* 47–55.

Meredith, C., & Edworthy, J. (1995). Are there too many alarms in the intensive care unit? An overview of the problems. *Journal of Advanced Nursing, 21,* 15–20.

Momtahan, K. L., Hetu, R., & Tansley, B. W. (1993). Audibility and identification of auditory alarms in operating rooms and an intensive care unit. *Ergonomics, 36,* 1159–1176.

Mylrea, K. C., Orr, J. A., & Westenskow, D. R. (1993). Integration of monitoring for intelligent alarms in anesthesia: Neural networks—can they help? *Journal of Clinical Monitoring, 9,* 31–37.

Navabi, M. J., Mylrea, K. C., & Watt, R. C. (1989). Detection of false alarms using an integrated anesthesia monitor. *IEEE Engineering Medical Biological Society 11th Annual International Conference, 11,* 1774–1775.

Orr, J. A., & Westenskow, D. R. (1994). A breathing circuit alarm system based on neural networks. *Journal of Clinical Monitoring, 10,* 101–109.

Seagull, F. J., & Sanderson, P. M. (2001). Anesthesia alarms in surgical context: An observational study. *Human Factors, 43*(1), 66–78.

Senders, J. W., & Moray, N. P. (1991). *Human error: Cause, prediction, and reduction.* Hillsdale, NJ: Lawrence Erlbaum Associates.

Stanton, N. A. (1994). Alarm initiated activities. In N. A. Stanton (Ed.), *Human factors in alarm design* (pp. 93–117). London: Taylor & Francis.

Topf, M., & Dillon, E. (1988): Noise-induced stress as a predictor of burnout in critical care nurses. *Heart Lung, 17,* 567–74.

Weinger, M. B. (1995). Cardiovascular reactivity among surgeons: Not music to everyone's ears. *Journal of the American Medical Association, 273,* 1090–1091.

Weinger, M. B., & Englund, C. E. (1990). Ergonomic and human factors affecting anesthetic vigilance and monitoring performance in the operating room environment. *Anesthesiology, 73,* 995–1021.

Woods, D. D. (1995). The alarm problem and directed attention in dynamic fault management. *Ergonomics, 38,* 2371–2394.

Xiao, Y., Hunter, W. A., Mackenzie, C. F., Jefferies, N. J., Horst, R., & the LOTAS Group (1996). Task complexity in emergency medical care and its implications for team coordination. *Human Factors, 38*(4), 636–645.

Xiao, Y., Mackenzie, C. F., Jaberi, M., Harper, B., & the LOTAS Group (1996). Alarms: Silenced, ignored, and missed. *Anesthesiology, 73,* 995–1021.

Xiao, Y., Mackenzie, C. F., Patey, R., & the LOTAS Group (1998). Team coordination and breakdowns in a real-life stressful environment. *Proceedings of the Human Factors and Ergonomics 42nd Annual Meeting, 1999* (pp. 186–190). Santa Monica, CA: Human Factors and Ergonomics Society.

Xiao, Y., & Seagull, F. J. (1999). An analysis of problems with auditory alarms: Defining the role of alarms in process monitoring tasks. *Proceedings of the Human Factors and Ergonomics Society 43rd Annual Meeting, 1999* (pp. 256–260). Santa Monica, CA: Human Factors and Ergonomics Society.

9 The Intensive Care Unit May Be Harmful to Your Health

Yoel Donchin
Hadassah Hebrew University
Medical Center

INTENSIVE CARE UNIT ATTENDING PHYSICIAN, WILLIAM JONES, M.D.

Dr. William Jones, the attending physician in the intensive care unit (ICU), works 5 days a week, is well paid, does not have to pay loans, and is in good health. His medical training was in anesthesia; he has had experience working in the ICU. He enters the ICU at 7 a.m. relaxed and confident to start another day. The minute he enters the ICU, he is exposed to its unique and noisy environment, the 10 patients he left just 12 hours ago, and the need to update himself on the condition of each of those patients plus the two who arrived in the ICU in the last hour. He begins to read the large amount of information on the patients' charts. The nurses are doing their rounds.

Within 5 minutes of Dr. Jones' arrival in the ICU, the radiology department requests the transfer of a patient for a computerized tomography (CAT scan) that must be organized immediately. He must complete his review of the charts and his evaluation of the medical condition of the each of the patients, be it stable, changed, or perhaps hopeless, in which case ethical measures must be taken. Based on the information from the charts, he issues new orders for the care of each patient. He has not finished issuing those orders when a call comes from the emergency room notifying him that a patient in critical condition is being sent for admission to the ICU. This presents a problem for Dr. Jones because criteria for admission of patients to the ICU are not well defined.

The broad screening criteria for admission states that patients should be accepted who are likely to die within 24 hours yet have a good chance of recovery if admitted to the ICU; however, no bed is available in the ICU for this new patient. Although beds frequently are made available for new patients by transferring ICU patients to standard hospital wards, from the information Dr. Jones has read during the brief time he has been on the ICU, there appears to be no clear candidate for transfer to a standard ward. Nonetheless, he gives the new patient a general examination to determine need for ICU care. After the examination and diagnosis, Dr. Jones negotiates an ICU bed for the new patient, records his orders on a special form specifying the manner of respiration, the rate of administration of fluids and medications, the posture in which to place the patient, special treatments, and requests for consultation and tests. The execution of the orders is the responsibility of the nursing team. Dr. Jones takes a deep breath and returns to issuing orders for treatment for the other ICU patients as he experiences the first pain of a migraine headache.

Thus even if a care provider arrives for work in a calm mood and good health, within a very short period the conditions in the ICU can cause overwhelming demands sometimes incompatible with human performance. Such demands can and do affect performance of care providers—performance that impacts patients, as in the case of Dr. Jacob Butcher.

Dr. Jacob Butcher was a successful surgeon in a local hospital not far from the capital city. He was the typical doctor as seen in the old movies. Like Dr. Ben Casey, he was hardworking and devoted to his patients. As he was reading one evening, with no warning, he suffered excruciating pain in his abdomen. He diagnosed himself as having pancreatitis; within 48 hours, he was admitted to the ICU of the hospital in which he practiced. Twenty-four hours later, he was transferred to the ICU of a major medical center. This is where our story begins. Unlike a classic detective story, I will disclose at the beginning how this story ends. Dr. Butcher was discharged from the hospital after a 3-month stay and currently is functioning normally.

When Jacob Butcher arrived as a patient at the ICU, he had a blue endotracheal tube in his mouth that was attached to a portable ventilator that pumped air into his lungs, thus breathing for him. Suspended above his head were seven different bags of fluids and drugs that he was receiving; all the plastic tubes leading the fluids of life into his veins were tangled on the bed. Locating the origin of each plastic tube required the expertise of a weaver; Nurse Roth managed to unravel the tangle. Because the automatic syringes that controlled the flow of medications were not in use during the ambulance transport, it was necessary to verify which tube was connected to what bag.

    The bags contained some drugs in concentrations that were not used in this particular ICU, so it was necessary to prepare the proper dose. Nurse Bates added 2 ampoules of Dopamine, a drug administered to maintain blood pressure and strengthen the heart muscle, to the 500 ml of saline, as was the usual practice. From this bag, she filled 200 ml into a special reservoir that protects the patient from getting too much fluids or drug. She removed the bag from the referral hospital, substituted the one she had prepared, and attached it to the intravenous (IV) infusion pump, a computer-chip-based device that is programmed to regulate the flow of fluids by controlling the drops. Ten minutes later, Dr. Butcher's blood pressure rose to 190 and his heart rate accelerated to 166—both abnormally high. The alarms on the monitors sounded, indicating something was wrong. To the nurse's surprise, the 200-ml container of Dopamine that was to be administered slowly during 20 hours ran out within minutes. This was a new model of the infusion device that looked the same as the older models but was programmed differently. After the drug was discontinued, Dr. Butcher's heart rate went down to normal and his blood pressure returned to its previous value. During this time, he was fully sedated with an intravenous drug and did not feel a thing.

    Later in the afternoon, Dr. Butcher's lab results came in; they were very strange. His BUN, the level of urea in the blood that reflects the functioning of the kidneys, was three times higher than the previous reading from the referral hospital. His potassium reading was at a level almost incompatible with life. Mr. David Blecher in Bed 2, a patient with chronic renal failure, received the best lab results ever—namely, normal BUN and normal potassium. This was not due to the care he received; rather it indicated a mix-up of names when labeling the test tubes containing specimens from the two patients.

    There were no more alarming events on the first night; however, during the morning rounds, Dr. Butcher's chart indicated he was not producing enough urine. A fluid load (increase) was immediately ordered. Later, when the nurse from the morning shift recalculated the total urine output using a calculator, unlike the night shift nurse who had done all the calculations in her tired head, she realized that 2.450 + 1230 does not equal 1213. The physician on duty promptly cancelled his order for the extra fluids.

    A few days later, the oxygen saturation level, as measured from the tip of the finger via a pulse oximeter (an optic, noninvasive detector) fell from 99% to 84%, which was an alarming sign. Dr. Butcher's chest x-ray was normal; the endotracheal tube was placed in the proper position through his mouth to his lungs enabling ventilation. A careful physical examination revealed no abnormal findings. The team on the afternoon shift discussed a few theories about the causes of the low oxygen saturation reading for Dr. Butcher.

    On a routine check, the respiratory therapist discovered that the oxygen concentration knob, a small, almost unrecognizable, knob on the wall oxygen outlet, a knob lacking any safety features to avoid unintentional position change, was not at the proper setting. Without saying a word, he set it to the correct position and Dr. Butcher's saturation level returned to normal. The problem with the knob confirmed what the medical staff had been trying to communicate to the hospital administration—that the oxygen outlets on the walls are old and can cause problems; they are accidents waiting to happen. The administration continued to state that it is too expensive to install new ones, so from time to time, an incident like this happens.

A very unusual event occurred on the 52nd day of Dr. Butcher's stay in the ICU. That event involved Osmolite, a special, tasteless nutrition solution that supplies necessary nutritional elements to the patient who cannot eat. Osmolite is fed via a nasogastric (NG) tube going from the mouth or nose into the patient's stomach. On this occasion, the bag containing the Osmolite that was to go into Dr. Butcher's stomach was inadvertently substituted for the IV nutrition solution that was connected to a tube inserted into the patient's central vein instead of the NG tube. At the last minute, the head nurse, who just happened to be passing by, noticed this and avoided a very serious incident.

Throughout Dr. Butcher's stay in the ICU until he left the unit, there were more potential incidents. For example, some drugs continued to be administered for a few days after orders to discontinue them had been given. This was discovered on one occasion at the beginning of an afternoon shift when Dr. Ben, the resident during the morning shift, said he thought he had ordered discontinuing a particular drug; the nurse on duty swore that she had never received that order. There was no time to determine why the confusion happened because rounds were resumed in response to pressure to release the morning team so they would not miss their ride on the transportation provided by the hospital.

On another occasion, antibiotics were given twice. Fortunately, there were no adverse side effects. Other errors included administering too high and too low dosages of vasoactive drugs (medication that affects blood circulation), leaving a urinary catheter in place for 3 hours rather than a few minutes, and failing to diagnose pneumothorax (a common complication of ventilated patients where air enters the tissues surrounding the lungs and disturbs ventilation unless it is evacuated via a chest drain), which can be easily diagnosed through chest x-rays. Fortunately, most of the errors were discovered before they caused any real damage and what did happen had no lasting affect, so Dr. Butcher survived his stay in the ICU.

Is this a true story? The patient is real. All of the events actually did occur. Indeed, one to two potentially serious incidents per patient per day in the ICU are attributed to error (Donchin, Gopher, & Olin, 1995). If not discovered in time, they could be fatal. Why is this rate so high? How can anyone survive? To answer these questions, let us consider the origin of the ICU and its evolution to the contemporary, technologically sophisticated ICU.

ORIGIN AND EVOLUTION OF THE ICU

The first person to propose that patients who had undergone surgery require specialized facilities and particularly dedicated care was Florence Nightingale, the legendary pioneering nurse (Smith, 1951). She recognized that the prevention of common complications resulting from surgery, namely vomiting and respiratory distress, necessitated the uninterrupted monitoring of postoperative patients. In her day, such monitoring could be accomplished only by intensive and constant personal surveillance. It required the meticulous and frequent checking of the patients' vital signs, such as the pulse rate, the character of the respiration, and color of the urine. The vigilance she proposed demanded a nursing staff specially trained to recognize, by sight and touch, the signs of postoperative distress. That component of competent, intensive care for the seriously ill patient stands in stark contrast to the type of intensive care that is provided today.

Acknowledgment of the need to gather all critical-care patients into one unit within the hospital followed the success of the individual pioneers who started resuscitating patients and treating severe diseases of the lung (Hall, Schmidt, & Wood, 1992). Initially, the ICU was a single room containing a respirator to ventilate patients who are unable to breathe, a monitor to record their heart rate, and most importantly, trained nurses to operate these complicated devices. In the first years following formal establishment of the ICU, the basic physiological and medical principles for treatment of critical patients were elaborated. Development of increasingly complicated surgical procedures that may last hours, such as open-heart and brain surgery, created the need for expanded supervision of patients, including intensive observation both during and post surgery.

Anesthesiologists were the first to apply their expertise to the ICU environment. This is reasonable because the patient in the operating room is basically in a one-bed ICU where the anesthesiologist provides intensive care for that patient during crucial moments of surgery. The anesthesiologist's responsibility for the patient's physiological integrity includes maintaining respiration by controlling the ventilator, blood pressure by regulating the flow of drugs, and temperature by using a heating mattress. By following their patients from the operating room to the ICU, it became possible for the anesthesiologists to continue to supervise their care in the postoperative period. In some hospitals, anesthesiologists who had become interested in the field assumed responsibility for the ICUs. In other hospitals, proactive surgeons left their operating rooms to establish ICU services. Physicians specializing in pulmonary physiology, as well as surgeons or anesthesiologists, depending on the initiative of the particular hospital, were appointed to supervise ICUs.

Specialized ICUs

As pressure to transfer patients from overburdened hospital wards to ICUs rapidly increased, specialized ICUs came into being to address the needs and requirements of various categories of patients and medical specialties. Neonatal ICUs care for premature newborns, usually in incubators; pediatric ICUs provide care for children from a few weeks of age to puberty. There are ICUs for the treatment of burn victims, ICUs for neurosurgical patients, and ICUs for patients suffering spinal injury. There also are ICUs that monitor patients admitted with acute myocardial infarction (heart attack) and those with arrhythmia (irregularities of the heart beat). All of the ICUs are equipped with sophisticated medical devices.

Sophisticated Medical Devices

To ensure that the sophisticated devices function optimally, technicians trained to service and maintain them are included in the staff of ICUs. In addition, the physical setting of the ICU is adapted to respond to the devices' needs for continuous supplies of medical gases, sterile water for dialysis, adequate electrical outlets and an uninterrupted supply of electricity, appropriate lighting, and a reduced level of noise. New areas of ICU specialization evolved within the various physician and nurse specialties. Those ICU specialist caregivers adapt to the conditions of the ICU by ingesting large amounts of information, much of which comes from sophisticated devices.

Information from Sophisticated Devices. It is crucial that the physician knows what drugs the patient is taking and understands the effect of such medication on the results of laboratory tests, as well as their influence on the heart, lungs, and blood vessels of the patient. The physician also must have access to all the data regarding the patient's on-going condition such as blood pressure, heart rate, urine output, body temperature, and much more. Can a human being with limited memory remember so many details, analyze all the possibilities, and arrive at a proper conclusion for the 6 to 12 ICU patients who must be treated simultaneously (Abramson, Wald, & Grenvik, 1980)? Before we answer this question, let us visit the ICU of a large, teaching hospital, the ICU in which Dr. Butcher was a patient. Please cover your clothes with the special ICU gown and shoe covering. Just press the code number on the door to open it and you are in.

VISIT TO AN ICU

As soon as we enter the ICU, we see 12 patients in special beds in a large room. The majority of patients in this ICU are postsurgery. There also are young patients who sustained major trauma and those who suffer from disease that damaged their ability to breathe—all in critical condition. The physical layout of ICUs is not uniform. In some hospitals, ICU patients occupy private rooms (cubicles); in others, patients occupy a large hall-like ward. The place where the medical staff actually provides intensive care to a patient, the standard working station of the ICU, consists of the patient's bed surrounded by an area approximately twice the size of the bed. This area contains the equipment required to monitor and treat the patient. This machine-dominated setting contrasts with that of the standard hospital ward, where the furniture surrounding the patient's bed accommodates the patient's personal needs.

Bed No. 6

Let us visit Bed No. 6. Although not a very human approach, patients are referred to by their bed number to simplify and expedite matters when conducting ICU rounds. As you can see in Fig. 9.1, equipment is placed both above and beside Bed No. 6; most of it is attached to electrical outlets in the adjacent wall. Patients in the ICU are dependent on life-sustaining machines that continuously pump potent drugs into their veins and artificially breathe for them. The various medical devices are mobile to facilitate the transfer of the patient to other locations within the hospital or within the ICU.

Equipment.   Above the bed is a machine that monitors the patient's vital signs. Data from various sensors located on the patient's skin or intrusively introduced into his blood vessels or heart are brought to a central screen that, as in an airplane cockpit, graphically displays the vital information. This information includes the tracking of the patient's cardiac status from an electrocardiogram (ECG) and graphic representations of the electronic measures of pressure in the arteries, the level of oxygen saturation in the blood measured by a pulse oximeter, the level of carbon dioxide in exhaled breath via capnography, and the body temperature. Additional devices such as the Swan-Ganz catheter that measures the filling pressure of the heart and a mixed venous saturation probe also may be present, thus increasing the information displayed on the screen. Although the monitor stores the data it gathers, nurses customarily use pencil and paper to record that information on a chart that is kept on or beside the patient's bed.

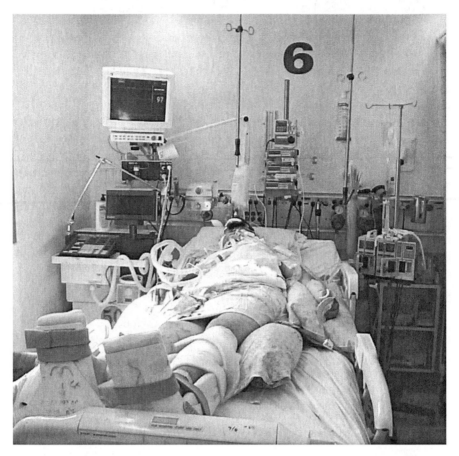

FIG. 9.1.   Bed 6 in the ICU at the Hadassah Hebrew University Hospital, Jerusalem, Israel.

Equipment located at the bedside falls into two categories: input equipment that supplies fluid and medications to the patient and output equipment that removes the patient's secretions from the stomach, chest, abdomen, and urinary tract. Also at the bedside in some cases, special equipment substitutes for or supports body functions such as a dialysis machine to substitute for a nonfunctional kidney and haemofiltration equipment to purify the blood from an overdose of drugs or dangerous levels of electrolytes in the blood, or a balloon pump to support a failing heart. These devices are attached to the patient with tubes and to wall outlets by electrical cables. There may be as many as 30 tubes exiting and entering a patient's body.

A wall outlet near the patient's bed in the ICU supplies both oxygen and compressed air to allow the preparation of different concentrations of oxygen to be administered to the patient via the respirator. Plastic tubes carry the mixture of oxygen and air from the outlet into the patient's lungs via pressure generated by the respirator. Many electrical outlets that provide power for the various medical devices also are on the wall. As all the tubes and wires are gathered at the same location—the patient—they intermingle like macaroni, hence the unofficial term *macaroni syndrome* as shown in Fig. 9.2.

Augmenting the harshness of the setting is the presence of an alarm that beeps and a light that flashes on each piece of equipment. The alarms sound at a rate of 1 to 5 per minute. In a six-bed ICU with many alarms sounding simultaneously, the noise can be irritating and identifying the source of an alarm can be difficult. In addition to the numerous, sometimes noisy machines and the plethora of tubes, cables, flashing lights, and beeping alarms, strong lighting in the ICU is mandatory 24 hours a day. A conscious patient, surrounded by the cacophony of ICU sounds that resemble white noise and the relentless light, can experience a form of sensory deprivation that is manifest as ICU psychosis. The congested and overwhelmingly artificial work setting, as well as the small area

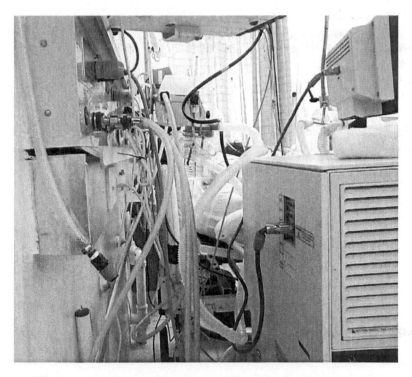

FIG. 9.2.   The *macaroni syndrome* of tubes and wires from a patient's medical equipment.

surrounding the bed of the critical patient, is further taxed by the presence of nurses, physicians, and other allied personnel who need to access the patient, as well as members of the patient's family.

ICU MEDICAL STAFF

During hospitalization in the ICU, patients are treated by a large number of health care personnel: one or two nurses per bed and one to three attending physicians as well as the intensivist, the ICU specialist who is the ICU director and guides colleagues and residents as well as consultants. More nurses are needed for patients in separate cubicles. Physiotherapists, respiratory therapists, radiology technicians, and other technicians also may be part of the team.

ICU Nurse

Nursing care is a crucial part of the ICU. The nurses not only carry the main burden of the daily work, but they also are responsible for the continuity of memory about the patients and the uninterrupted transfer of information about the day-to-day changes within the unit as well as the follow-up of the critically ill. Without the nurses, there is no intensive care. Technology without experienced nurses has absolutely no value. Nurses in the ICU are assigned to specific patients, usually to one or sometimes two patients, unlike the physician who is responsible for 10 to 20 patients at a time. Although there are official ICU nursing procedures, the dynamics of intensive care inevitably prompts many deviations.

In addition to executing the physician's orders, the ICU nurse is responsible for collecting and recording information about the patient such as respiratory rate, which is measured by using an instrument as well as by direct observation. The nurse must keep abreast of many parameters on the monitors: the heart rate and the shape of the ECG, the blood pressure waveform, the central venous pressure, body temperature, and oxygenation, to name only a few. When required, the nurse must respond immediately and must record and date in the patient's chart all the data generated by the monitors; the nurse also is responsible for ensuring that the potent medications used in the ICU are administered in precise dosages. Any deviation can be dangerous to the patient.

ICU AS THE TEMPLE OF TECHNOLOGY

The hospital ICU is dedicated to the care of the seriously ill patient. ICUs typically are equipped with the most advanced medical technology and are intended to provide patients with the best medical care available. Nevertheless, care in the

ICU has been found to expose patients to substantial risk resulting from the limited ability of the persons working in this environment to cope with both the technology and the enormous amount of data presented to them. To respond to a change in the medical condition of each patient, as in the case of Dr. Butcher, the attending physician must have access to the patient's medical history, which often is very long and complicated.

Impact of Technology

Contemporary caregivers are required to know the patient primarily as a set of numbers and laboratory results. Part of the daily care of the patient involves routine nursing procedures that make the difference between an ICU and a regular ward. Although it is the continuity of care that is of the utmost importance, the medical staff needs to simultaneously observe both the trends of the data and the patient's appearance and mental condition. It is absolutely necessary to pay strict attention to details that escape the monitoring system and can only be detected by good, old-fashioned, clinical observation. No monitor or device will supply information regarding a red irritation or reaction at the site of an infusion. There is no substitute for the meticulous observation of the patient's skin; only a clinician can discover that the patient is waking up from a deep coma. Nonetheless, the emphasis is on information provided by technologically sophisticated medical devices and tests.

Not only do the demands of technologically supplied information restrict the time available for clinical observations, but the continuous flow of data which must be integrated with other data such as laboratory test results, background information, previous diagnosis, care plan, and medication can cause information overload. That overload results in an inability to efficiently use all of the information available about the patient's state (Sukuvaara & Koski, 1995).

Whereas the early caregivers had to observe, talk to, and touch patients to stay abreast of their health status, today's ICU caregivers mainly refer to data provided by the technologically sophisticated devices that monitor patients. ICU personnel familiarize themselves with the physiological status of patients such as heart regularity from the ECG, blood pressure from invasive intra-arterial cannulae (tubes placed in an artery), and the qualities of the blood from the sophisticated flow-directed balloon as well as the Swan-Ganz catheter. Despite its importance, interaction between the medical staff and the patient is purely a matter of personal preference constrained by available time.

Physical Environment

The physical environment of the ICU can be detrimental to optimal care (Donchin et al., 1995). The area around the patient's bed is congested by instruments, monitors, wires, and IV lines. This often complicates access to the patient's head, which creates problems of identification and status assessment as well as airway access in case of a rapid change in condition. Means of providing care such as tubes, fluid bags, and drugs typically are insufficiently marked or have labels that are difficult to read (Donchin et al., 1995). The forms for recording information often are not designed specifically for the needs of the ICU, which forces many staff members to improvise and develop their own style. Other forms can be inappropriate in terms of layout and clarity of display.

Stress

The medical staff in the ICU works under considerable stress due to the harsh time constraints imposed by the immediacy of the patient's condition. They must wage a constant battle to preempt the development of ever more urgent conditions such as hemorrhaging and cardiac failure, and to prevent the rapid deterioration of the patient's condition due to severe sepsis. Sepsis, a life-threatening infection, is the most dangerous threat to the life of the patient today. Microbes are very efficient and formidable foes.

It is not possible to converse with most patients in the ICU as they are either heavily sedated, under the influence of medication, or they need to be mechanically ventilated by a respirator which breathes for them, as in the case of Dr. Butcher. Being ventilated prevents a patient from talking because air from the respirator travels via the endotracheal tube bypassing the vocal chords. For those patients who cannot verbally describe what is wrong or regulate their fluid intake and urine output, the ICU physician, the intensivist, must use readings from various monitoring devices to serve as those patients' regulatory functions.

The ICU patient's physiological vital signs displayed on the monitor can change at a very rapid pace; it is crucial to discover such changes as soon as they take place. For example, in the ICU it is essential to follow the patient's blood pressure from second to second. As a pilot in the cockpit must continuously observe the instruments that provide vital flight data, the ICU medical staff must continuously observe the monitors of their patients' vital signs. This is in contrast to internal medicine ward patients for whom physiological changes typically are so gradual that it is acceptable to measure blood pressure every 6 hours.

The rapid pace of gathering data for diagnostic purposes is characteristic of the activities in the ICU, such as the daily recording of more than 30 important parameters. These include all the measurements taken by the nurse, from the blood pressure and heart rate to the hourly output of urine. The ability of the personnel to respond on short notice to the rapidly changing condition of the patient requires the prompt analysis of the data and the swift execution of tests and other related activities. Orders written on admission of the patient to the ICU may be invalid within a brief period. The ICU physician needs and expects test results immediately, whereas the physician in the internal medicine ward is satisfied to receive the results of tests taken in the morning in time for the evening rounds. In the ICU, consultation with specialists occurs as soon as the need is identified. Prompt and appropriate responses to changes in the patient's condition are necessary to avoid further deterioration (Sexton, Thomas, & Helmreich, 2000).

Technological developments have occurred to meet the need for immediate test results. A machine the size of a small television set has been created that, when stationed within the ICU and operated by members of the ICU team, can provide results of electrolytes and blood gases in a matter of minutes from the analysis of a few drops or a teaspoon of blood. That machine, the blood gas analyzer (BGA), has revolutionized postoperative patient care. Rather than sending blood samples to various laboratories in the hospital and waiting hours to get the results, the patient's haemodynamic status (the condition of the heart and circulation), oxygen concentration in the blood, the level of acidity in the tissues, as well as lung and kidney functions, can be accurately ascertained within a few minutes using the BGA.

Technology and Stress.   Staff in the ICU function under considerable stress, pressured by time constraints imposed by the immediacy of patients' needs and the battle to preempt the natural progression of urgent conditions such as rapid deterioration due to severe sepsis, hemorrhage, and cardiac failure. In addition, the work environment is noisy and crowded—conditions that cause stress. It is increasingly acknowledged that traditional ICU working conditions impose an untenable degree of mental and physical stress on the medical personnel who staff them; such stress undermines the quality of care that they are able to provide. Much of the stress has been traced to the actual physical environment in which intensive care is administered.

The rapid, spontaneous development of intensive care technology over the past 40 years has generated an extraordinarily harsh environment that is incompatible with the human needs of health care personnel. The dedicated caregivers who initiated intensive care could not have anticipated the direction that management of critical patients would take. Their successors, captivated by the evolving potential of technological devices to save or prolong lives, are oblivious to the increasingly alienating work environment that rampant technology has been creating for providers of intensive care.

Communication

Nurses in the ICU are assigned to specific patients. Work in the ICU is carried out in three shifts, and each change of shift requires transfer of a great deal of detailed information about the patients. The content of that information is vital to the course and outcome of patient care, so effective communication and transfer of information between doctors and nurses is critical (Donchin et al., 1995). Nurses have closer and more continuous monitoring of each patient than do physicians. By serving as an active liaison, they can help doctors bridge information gaps and avoid confusion.

In the training environment, proper communication and exchange patterns can enable residents and students in the unit to learn conventions and routines from the accumulated experience of nurses. Often, however, a lack of effective information exchange in verbal communications occurs between ICU physicians and nurses. This has been a factor in one third of reported errors (Donchin et al., 1995). This is surprisingly high considering that verbal communications between physicians and nurses were observed only in 2% of the activities.

The Human Factor

About 40 years after the introduction of technological monitoring in ICUs, attention has turned to the human beings who provide care in the intensive care environment and how that environment may affect them. It was only after the best pilots of the Royal Air Force in England demonstrated an alarming degree of fatigue and incompetence that a thorough examination of the cockpit was conducted. Factors that contributed to those conditions were identified and many necessary changes were made. A similar examination of the conditions in the ICU finds error-provoking factors.

The reality is that ICU caregivers are social beings. Although they appreciate the value of the information readily produced by the various inanimate, technologically sophisticated devices on which their attention must be focused, their minimal human needs are not met in the pervasively artificial setting of the modern ICU. To meet those needs as well as reduce the likelihood of error through miscommunication, it is necessary to create an atmosphere of continuous communication between the different teams. Until that occurs, the ICU that gave life to so many people may be dangerous to the patients.

ICU AS A LABORATORY

The ICU may be considered as a large laboratory because the continuous monitoring and meticulous recording of critically ill patients' functioning allows the examination of those patients' responses to drugs and the immediate physiological effects of treatment. For example, physiological measurements done in the ICU and in the laboratory demonstrate that during the state of shock, there is no blood supply to the tissues, and adding drugs that cosmetically increase blood pressure contributes to deepening the deleterious effect of shock. As a result of that better understanding of the mechanism of shock, physicians are more tolerant of short periods of hypovelomic shock or low blood pressure due to bleeding, and administer blood and fluid to restore blood pressure rather than a drug to force a higher value. Indeed, because of this better understanding of shock, use of medications such as Isoproterenol to increase blood pressure has been withdrawn.

Based on the ability to accurately measure on-going physiological parameters, the physician is able to discover and respond to signs of deterioration in the patient's condition by providing logical and supportive treatment before it is too late. Hence, intensive care has become increasingly proactive. By measuring and recording, every hour, the patient's urine output as well as the volume of clear fluids and other intake such as food and drugs, it is possible to accurately balance and repair any deficit by increasing or withholding the fluid administration every few hours. Working in the ICU has been compared to the work of a pilot and to that of an air traffic controller. Although there is no basis for comparison of tasks, the level of responsibility—that of caring for the lives of others—is similar, as is the potential for error and the dire consequences of mistakes occurring in these highly charged circumstances.

ERROR

It was clear from our visit to the ICU that the physical setting of the ICU and its accouterments are not friendly to the medical team and are likely to contribute to error. For example, illegible print on IV bags presents, in a similar uniform manner, important information as well as unimportant details required by law. Even on close scrutiny, deciphering whether a solution contains 5% or 15% glucose is difficult. This is dangerous because administering 15% glucose to a patient with high blood sugar may have very deleterious consequences. Similarly, the identification of containers of potassium that could cause considerable damage to patients is not clear. Strict regulations regarding the storage of potassium were developed to avoid the fatal consequences of the erroneous administration of this dangerous drug. Despite best efforts by ICU personnel, errors can occur.

More errors per hour occur during the day than at night because more active care and procedures are performed during the day, hence more opportunities for error. When taking into account the typical instability of the medical status of ICU patients and the complex and demanding task of physicians and nurses, an overall error rate lower than 0.5% percent, of which only 29% were rated severe (Donchin et al., 1995), may be considered a very high and reliable level of performance. Given the critical condition of the patients and the large number of daily activities per patient, the percentages compute to two errors with the potential for a severe adverse outcome per patient per day. This is a matter of concern.

It is not surprising that in the 1980s, reports about mistakes in the ICU began to appear in literature describing the stress experienced by ICU staff (Merrill & Boisaubin, 1981). The most common errors reported were related to the administering of medications. (Tissot et al., 1999). Although this indicated an urgent need for a major research initiative to identify factors that contribute to error, fear of legal prosecution for admitting to errors inhibited its development.

HIGH VISIBILITY—HIGH COST

Hospital administrators have mixed feelings regarding the ICU. On one hand, it is the flagship of the hospital, the place to bring the mayor or other distinguished guests. It is also the temple of technology, the pride of the organization. On the other hand, the costs of maintaining an ICU are extremely high. When the hospital management wants to lower expenses, a good place appears to be the ICU. For example, the number of nurses at the evening shift might be reduced; however, such intervention is likely to decrease the effectiveness of the ICU.

If instead of one nurse per patient, the ratio is increased to one nurse per 1.5 patients, not only will the quality of care be different, but the workload will be heavier and the team more prone to errors. It is no wonder that in order to perform the 1,001 tasks for which nurses are responsible, they will try shortcuts that may work only part of the time. Attempts to cut costs in the design of a new ICU are also not realistic because it is very difficult to design a new ICU in an old building. The ICU requires space, personnel, and money.

ICU Ethical Dilemma

Controversy continues to rage regarding issues such as the criteria for admission of patients to the ICU, for ceasing treatment of critical patients, and for initiating or withholding treatment in the first place. The average length of stay in the ICU is from 4 to 7 days; Dr. Butcher's stay was exceptionally long. The ICU mortality rate of 20% would be considered extremely high for a regular hospital ward. That 20% mortality rate for an ICU, however, means that instead of a 100% mortality rate for 100 critically ill patients who would die without ICU care, 80 are saved; only 20 die. This underscores the importance of the ICU.

The rapid pace of unchecked technological development that enables prolonging life by maintaining some patients on a ventilator for years raises ethical issues that the medical establishment did not anticipate and for which they are not prepared. The ethical dimension of critical care has been elaborated, analyzed, and well documented (Oppenheim & Sprung, 1998; Sprung, Eidelman, & Pizov, 1997). Indeed, medical ethics has become field of study in its own right. Nonetheless, profound ethical questions confront ICU personnel.

Should a cancer patient without hope for improvement be maintained on a ventilator? Would that prolong the patient's life or misery? A diagnosis of brain death authorizes disconnecting a patient from the ventilator; however, a family that refuses to have the patient disconnected could keep a young person who might be saved with ICU care from being admitted because that ICU bed is unavailable. Should a patient with no hope of surviving be sent to the department of internal medicine where supervision is not as meticulous as in the ICU? Should a few more monitors be purchased or the budget stretched to hire more nurses who are more beneficial to the patient but more expensive (Nyman & Sprung, 1997)?

CONCLUSION

Health care providers have become accustomed to the encroachment of technology; however, people entering an ICU for the first time as visitors may feel they have entered the control room of a nuclear power plant where technology dominates. After a few moments, they observe that human beings are connected to all those wires and understand they are in a hospital—a place where technology and medicine are working together.

The ICUs of hospitals are locations dedicated to the care of the seriously ill patient. Typically, ICUs are equipped with the most advanced medical technology and are intended to provide patients with the best medical care available. Nevertheless, care in the ICU has been found to expose patients to a substantial risk resulting from human error. For example, unintentional disconnection of the endotracheal tube from the ventilator will stop the patient's breathing and cause irreparable damage; therefore, every machine is equipped with alarms to alert others to this unfortunate event. Because of the number of machines that alarm and because most alarms sound the same, it is often difficult to identify the device emitting the alarm, which can delay correcting the problem.

The development of advanced technology has been the primary focus of efforts to provide the best care possible to critically ill patients in the ICU, but the human factor has been greatly neglected. It is increasingly acknowledged that traditional ICU working conditions impose an untenable degree of mental and physical stress on the medical personnel who staff the facilities. The source of much of the stress has been traced to the actual physical environment in which intensive care is administered (Donchin et al., 1995). This stress undermines the quality of care that they are able to provide.

The physical environment also can stress the patients if they are conscious. To provide quality care, the medical staff must be acutely conscious, which heightens the impact of the conditions of the ICU, their work setting, on them. The rapid development of intensive care technology has produced an extraordinarily demanding environment that is incompatible with the human needs of health care personnel as they provide treatment for the sickest of patients. Thus, the ICU that has given life to so many people may be harmful to the care providers as well as the patients.

REFERENCES

Abramson, N. S., Wald, K. S., & Grenvik, A. N. A. (1980). Adverse occurrences in intensive care units. *Journal of the American Medical Association, 244,* 1582–1584.

Donchin, Y., Gopher, D., & Olin, M. (1995) A look into the nature and causes of human error in the intensive care unit. *Critical Care Medicine, 5:23*(2), 294–300.

Hall, J. B., Schmidt, G. A., & Wood, L. D. H. (1992). The origin and evolution of critical care: Editorial introduction. In *Principles of critical care* (pp. xxxxi–xxxviii). New York: McGraw Hill.

Merrill, J. M., & Boisaubin, E. V. (1981). Adverse occurrence in the intensive care unit. *Journal of the American Medical Association, 27:245*(12), 1214–1215.

Nyman, D. L., & Sprung, C. L. (1997) International perspective on ethics in critical care. *Critical Care Clinics, 13*(2), 409–415.

Oppenheim, A., & Sprung, C. L. (1998). Cross-cultural ethics decision-making in critical care (editorial comment). *Critical Care Medicine, 26*(3), 447–451.

Sexton, J. B., Thomas, E. J., & Helmreich, R. L. (2000). Error, stress and team work in medicine and aviation: Cross sectional surveys. *British Medical Journal, 320,* 745–749.

Smith, C. W. (1951). *Florence Nightingale 1820–1910.* New York: McGraw Hill.

Sprung, C. L., Eidelman, L., & Pizov, R. (1997). Ethics and the law in intensive care medicine. *Acta Anaesthesioloica Scandanavica* Suppl.; *111,* 160.

Sukuvaara, T., & Koski, E. M. J. (1995). Informative alarms in anaesthesia: From signal to patient-state monitoring. *Current Opinion in Anaesthesia, 8*(6), pp. 526–531.

Tissot, E., Cornette, C., Demoley, P., Jacquet, M., Barale, F., & Capellier, G. (1999). Medication errors at the administration stage in an intensive care unit. *Intensive Care Medicine, 25*(4), 353–359.

10 Challenges and Adverse Events in the Home

Denise M. Korniewicz
University of Miami School of Nursing

Maher El-Masri
University of Windsor, Ontario, Canada

HOME HEALTH NURSE, MRS. JEAN LOWE, R.N.

Mrs. Jean Lowe, R.N., completed her baccalaureate degree in nursing a year ago. She had been working as a home health aide for 3 years when she decided to become a registered nurse. She needed a stable income; she received minimal child support from her ex-husband for her children ages 12, 14, and 16. Registered nurses were making over $50,000, so Jean, at 35 years of age, pursued her degree and professional licensure for the financial security needed to assist her children with college. It took several years to complete the degree because it was necessary for her to work while she attended classes. Because she had worked as a home health aide for so long, Jean felt confident in her home care clinical practice skills and knowledge after her licensure so she joined a private for-profit home care nursing company (WECARE) in San Diego.

Because WECARE Home Health Nursing Services was known among nurses to pay substantially higher hourly rates than other companies, Jean found she could double her income through extra overtime by working 12-hour shifts 6 days a week. Although her paychecks were substantial, Jean found that after she paid for her children's needs, the mortgage, living expenses, and college investment plans she had little left. There was a major nursing shortage so she had the opportunity to supplement her income by working seven 12- or 16-hour shifts at least twice a month, which she did.

Four months after she joined WECARE, it merged with another home health company and started providing contractual services for three times the number of patients. Immediately after the merger, the service was so busy that the existing nursing staff was offered financial bonuses to work 16-hour shifts, especially on weekends. Jean, being an experienced nurse and previously a home health aide, signed up for weekly extra hours in addition to her 7-day work plans. She knew that the agency needed her and that any hours she agreed to work would be well compensated financially.

After working 7 consecutive days of 12- or 16-hour shifts, Jean decided to work a 16-hour shift on the 8th consecutive day, Saturday, and take Sunday off for her son's birthday. On Saturday, Jean began her day by reporting to the agency at 7 a.m. when she obtained her assignment. The agency supervisor knew that Jean was experienced and scheduled her for 12 patients, with eight of them requiring at least an hour of nursing care during the visit. Armed with her patient load, Jean prioritized her care and decided to visit the eight more acute patients before the others. If she arrived at her last patient's house by 9 p.m., she knew it would be a reasonable hour for the family. She allowed the last hour of her shift for completing paperwork at the office.

Jean left the nursing agency by 7:30 a.m.; she arrived at her first patient, Mrs. Tindell, by 8 a.m. and her day began. Mrs. Tindell was recently discharged after a 72-hour stay in the hospital, which included colostomy surgery (bowel resection with feces collected into an attached bag) and recovery time. Apparently, Mrs. Tindell was not instructed on the proper care of her colostomy, changing procedures, or use of medical supplies during her hospital stay because she thought she needed to change the whole colostomy set every time she had a bowel movement or whenever feces were in the bag. She had used the entire month's supply of bags and other medical supplies in far less than a month. Because Mrs. Tindell did not follow the proper procedures for applying the stoma adhesive (adhesive to attach the bag to the opening in the bowel), she was experiencing leakage from the colostomy. Jean also noted that the skin was bleeding around the stoma site and it seemed to be spurting blood. Jean knew this was abnormal so she phoned Mrs. Tindell's physician, Dr. Han, and left a message to have her call returned.

Jean cleaned the stoma site and instructed the patient about when to change the colostomy bags, how to do proper skin care, and approximately how many times a day the colostomy bag would need to be changed. It was now 9 a.m. and Dr. Han had not called back. When Jean phoned the medical supply company authorized by Mrs. Tindell's Health Maintenance Organization (HMO) for replacement supplies, she was told it was closed on Saturdays and would not be open until Monday. The supplies were urgently needed, so Jean immediately began calling other medical supply companies; however, none would send the supplies because the HMO had already authorized a 1-month supply. Therefore, Jean had to contact the hospital and request delivery of the supplies to meet Mrs. Tindell's needs until Monday when the medical supply company could provide them. Arranging for the stopgap supplies took Jean over 1½ hours.

Jean continued to request that Dr. Han be paged. Finally, she received a call from Dr. Han's answering service stating that he was on vacation and one of his partners would return her call. Fifteen minutes later, Dr. Han's partner, Dr. James, called. Jean reported the unusual bleeding; Dr. James suggested that she attach a pressure bandage and tell Mrs. Tindell to come to his office on Monday morning. Jean explained that this was highly unusual bleeding and that she did not think a pressure dressing would be enough. She suggested that Dr. James see Mrs. Tindell at the local emergency department. Dr. James, who did not know Mrs. Tindell, did not think that was necessary. He instructed Jean to have the family observe Mrs. Tindell and if the bleeding did not stop, take her to the emergency room where the emergency room doctor could call him if it was warranted. Jean hung up the telephone and instructed the family according to her conversation with Dr. James. It was now 10 a.m.; Jean left for the next patient's house 20 minutes away. En route, she began to estimate her time because she had 11 more patients to care for during her 16-hour shift.

Jean arrived at Mr. Smith's home at 10:30 a.m. Mr. Smith recently was discharged after being hospitalized for an acute myocardial infarction (heart attack) with chronic congestive heart failure. When Jean entered the house, she noticed that Mrs. Smith was quite anxious. Jean asked what was wrong; Mrs. Smith gestured for Jean to come to her husband's room. Once Jean entered the room she noticed that Mr. Smith was extremely cyanotic (blue), gasping for breath, and unable to respond to questions. The nasal cannula (the oxygen tube that provides air to the patient via two nasal prongs) was in place but there was no oxygen flow and the pressure gauge on the oxygen tank indicated it was empty. When Jean asked Mrs. Smith if she knew the tank was empty and how long it had been reading empty, the wife replied, "I didn't know what it meant and I knew you were coming today so I decided to wait since I was not sure what to do."

Jean assessed Mr. Smith by checking his breathing, blood pressure, and lungs. She noted that he was having difficulty breathing because his lungs were filled with fluid caused by his congestive heart failure. Jean immediately called an ambulance to transfer him to the emergency room. Unfortunately, there was no oxygen cylinder to oxygenate him while waiting for the ambulance. Apparently, the hospital discharge nurse did not contact the medical respiratory supply company to deliver oxygen regularly. By the time the paramedics arrived, Mr. Smith was on the verge of a respiratory arrest. Jean told the paramedics about Mr. Smith's condition, instructed Mrs. Smith to accompany her husband to the hospital, and noted that it took the ambulance service over 30 minutes to respond. Jean secured the house, documented the incident, and proceeded on to her next patient.

It was now noon and Jean was worried about completing the remaining 10 patients assigned for the day. To catch up, Jean decided to skip lunch and drive to her third patient, approximately 30 minutes away. She called the family to inform them of the delay. They were upset because she was already a few hours late; however, they told her to come anyway. The route she normally took was under repair; it was Saturday, so a portion of the road was closed to traffic. The detour was an extra 3 miles out of the way which, although she drove as quickly as possible, made her later than expected. Jean arrived at 1 p.m. and was met by the patient's daughter Sue, who was angry that she had to wait so long. Jean apologized and proceeded to see the patient, Mrs. Kay.

Mrs. Kay was an obese 77-year-old patient with chronic congestive heart failure and arthritis, who was authorized an airflow bed to prevent her from getting pressure sores. Most recently, Mrs. Kay had had abdominal surgery. Because the surgical wound was infected, it needed to heal from the inside to the outside, so the skin and fat of her wound remained open. Mrs. Kay required a lot of home care: wound dressing changes three times a day, monitored coughing and deep breathing, getting out of bed to sit in a chair, and a soft diet to assist in the healing process and faster rehabilitation. She also was receiving one week of intravenous (IV) antibiotics. After Jean assessed Mrs. Kay, she noted that the IV site was red and swollen, which kept the antibiotic from being infused. Jean also noted that the IV pump, which regulates the rate at which the fluid enters the vein, was not beeping to warn of the occlusion or fluid backup that had occurred. In addition, Jean noted that the airflow bed was not working properly— it was deflated and when she tried to reset the inflation button, it kept beeping and reading error.

Jean changed Mrs. Kay's dressing, gave her a bath (she had been incontinent), called the medical supply company for bed repairs, and instructed Mrs. Kay's daughter how to check the airflow bed, assess her mother's abdominal wound for changes, and how to move Mrs. Kay without injuring her own back. Mrs. Kay's daughter was very angry and stated that she was not interested in learning and expected the home health nurse(s) to provide whatever care her mother needed. Jean suggested that Mrs. Kay's daughter call other family members for assistance. It took Jean over an hour and a half to complete the nursing care required for Mrs. Kay. At 2:30 p.m. Jean left and proceeded on to her next patient, leaving her paperwork (documentation) for later.

Jean arrived to her fourth patient, Mr. Dee, by 3 p.m. and noted that although she had worked an 8-hour shift by that time, she had completed only one fourth of her patient assignment. She made a mental note to call her supervisor so that *additional help could be found to reassign some of her cases. At Mr. Dee's house Jean found such disarray that she thought it had been ransacked. Mrs. Dee was hiding in a corner, fearful and crying. She told Jean that her husband recently had been taken to the hospital for fainting. Upon hospital discharge, Mr. Dee was diagnosed with early stages of Alzheimer's disease. Although the information Jean had received included no indication of violent behavior by Mr. Dee, his wife had bruises on her arms, a black eye, and appeared totally exhausted from trying to care for her husband. It was apparent that Mrs. Dee was not informed about Alzheimer's disease and its progression.*

Mr. Dee was naked in the bedroom, dismantling the closet, throwing clothes and possessions about, and talking incessantly. When Mrs. Dee approached her husband, he slapped her across her face and pushed her into the bed. Jean tried to speak with Mr. Dee; however, he did not understand and swung at her with his cane. Jean decided that Mr. Dee obviously was having some type of violent dementia and phoned the social worker on call. In the meantime, Jean removed Mrs. Dee from the immediate area and secured her in another room. Jean went into Mr. Dee's room and tried to have him sit; however, he resisted and hit Jean across her face, causing her nose to bleed. Approximately 20 minutes later, the social worker called Jean back and instructed her to call the paramedics to transport Mr. Dee to the nearest emergency room for psychiatric evaluation and possible admission.

Jean found Mrs. Dee crouched in the corner crying and not sure what to do. Jean informed her that they were going to take Mr. Dee to the hospital, obtain some sedation, and try to admit him for further evaluation. Mrs. Dee refused to allow that to happen because she was worried that their HMO insurance would not pay for the emergency room coverage. She asked Jean to contact their primary care physician, Dr. Red. Jean did so and informed him of the situation. Dr. Red called back after contacting the Dees' HMO and instructed Jean to take Mr. Dee to an outpatient psychiatric walk-in service rather than the emergency department because the HMO policy required outpatient evaluation. Jean told Dr. Red that the paramedics were on the way and that the closest outpatient psychiatric service closed at noon on Saturday—it then was 3:45 p.m. She also told him that Mr. Dee could not be transported safely without sedation.

Because of the reimbursement constraints of the HMO, it was necessary for Dr. Red to refuse to authorize emergency treatment for Mr. Dee. He instructed Jean to have Mrs. Dee transport him to a 24-hour psychiatric outpatient treatment facility located 2 hours from their home. At this point, Jean was concerned about Mr. Dee's increasingly violent behavior and decided to ask her supervisor to call the health care agency's physician for authorization. Jean's supervisor called back within 30 minutes and told her to contact the paramedics for transportation to the nearest emergency room. Jean called the paramedics again,

*contacted Mrs. Dee's daughter to meet Mrs. Dee at the emergency room, and
began her routine documentation of the case. It was now 6 p.m. Jean began to
feel tired and hungry and she had eight more patients to see before 11 p.m.*

*After assessing the previous 8-hour-shift part of her day, Jean contacted her
home health agency supervisor to tell her that she was behind and to report her
shift to her. Jean expressed her frustration and told her supervisor that she'd to
deal with so many problems that she was not sure if she would be able to continue as a home health nurse. Jean's supervisor was sympathetic, saying that
some days she felt the same way; however, other days were not so bad. Jean's
supervisor reevaluated Jean's caseload and instructed her to complete two more
acute patients and report to the agency to complete her documentation. In the
meantime, because there were no other nurses available to reassign Jean's case
load, the supervisor prioritized the cases, contacted appropriate family members for the low priority cases, and told them they would not receive home health
services until the next day.*

ISSUES AND ADVERSE EVENTS

All the names and situations in the preceding story are fictitious; however, every
aspect of this narrative can and does occur in the practice of home health nursing
in agencies providing that care throughout the United States at the beginning of
the 21st century. The cases in the story illustrate risk factors associated with
adverse events and errors in health care and point to factors that plague patients
in need of health care services. The following discussion describes the growth of
home health care and errors in home health care.

Home Health Care

There were over 33.6 million admissions to U.S. hospitals in 1997 (American
Hospital Association [AHA], 2001), with well over 98,000 hospitalized Americans dying annually as a result of adverse events (Institute of Medicine, 1999).
The total costs (lost income, lost household production, disability and health
care costs) of preventable adverse events (medical errors resulting from injury)
are estimated to be between $17 and $29 billion, half of which is the actual cost
of health care necessitated by those events (Thomas, Studdert, & Newhouse,
1999). These figures represent only hospitalized patients; they do not include
patients who are cared for in the community, nursing homes, assisted living
homes, who live with and are cared for by relatives, or who receive services from
home health agencies.

Although more and more care is being provided in out-patient settings such
as ambulatory surgical facilities, physician offices, and clinics, adverse events

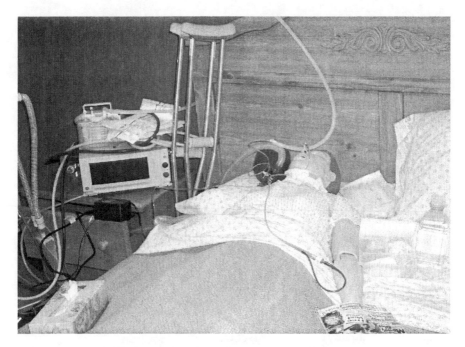

FIG. 10.1.   View of complicated equipment in the home.

related to these settings have not been well documented; essentially, such information is not available. Most efforts related to adverse events have focused on hospitals; however, medical errors present a problem in any setting. In home care, where patients and family members are required to use complicated equipment, assess patient needs, and perform often-complicated follow-up care, the risk of error and adverse health outcomes is even greater than in hospitals or outpatient settings. A rather typical home care setting is illustrated in Fig. 10.1. Note the cluttered area, which could result in a patient injury.

Initially, home health care nursing practice took the form of private or visiting nurses. A private nurse literally lived in the patient's house and dealt with the patient and family with day-to-day activities. Nurses who lived in these situations often found it difficult to separate their personal lives from their professional lives. The community did not value nurses in the home setting and viewed them as servants (Haddad & Kapp, 1991). With the revolution in nursing education and the growth of the feminist movement in the 20th century, nursing moved toward the hospital settings, and the image of the nurse started to change within society. Additionally, the American Nurses Association (ANA) endorsement of home health certification (Chusid, 1987; Joel, 1989) changed the image of the home health nurse to that of a professional who manages not one but many patients at one time. During the last two decades, home health nursing practice has expanded beyond the traditional style of home care to include age-related groups (such as the elderly) and more acutely ill patients.

As health care changed with the coming of managed care, services have become decentralized and fragmented. The social values related to these changes and their impact on safe patient care have not been questioned by consumers (Hellinghausen, 1999); however the impact is profound as patients are discharged in a subacute state, a state that requires substantial home care as illustrated by the patients cared for by Jean Lowe in the story. Home health nursing care is a fertile environment for the study of factors that contribute to human error and patient adverse events. There is little in the literature specifically related to home health nursing and adverse events; rather, there are data about risk factors associated with home health nursing such as infection control, home safety, environmental considerations, uses of medical devices, and their impact on patient outcomes. Home health nursing practice is linked with health care organizations that provide comprehensive and continual patient care services. Due to changes brought about by HMOs and managed care, such as reimbursement being keyed to diagnosis rather than the type and quality of patient care being rendered, delivery of health care is fragmented and lacks tracking methods to provide information pertaining to the continuity of care (Chassin & Gavin, 1998).

FACTORS ASSOCIATED WITH ADVERSE EVENTS IN HOME HEALTH NURSING CARE

A number of factors affected Jean's ability to provide effective, quality nursing care and safe clinical practice. Fragmentation, poor communication, inadequate medical supplies, lack of patient teaching, and limited hospital stays all contributed to the difficulties Jean experienced in attempting to provide home nursing care. Major categories of factors that affect the quality of home health care nursing services and contribute to error are infection control, reimbursement, communication, the nursing shortage, and the use of technology.

The Importance of Infection Control

As a nurse, Mrs. Jean Lowe assessed infection control issues in each of her patients by noting the environment: infection control issues including general overall assessment, dressing changes, skin integrity, surgical site, and IV site, and complications associated with commonly acquired infections. Jean was instrumental in teaching the family members about the prevention, signs, and symptoms associated with an infection and follow-up treatment options.

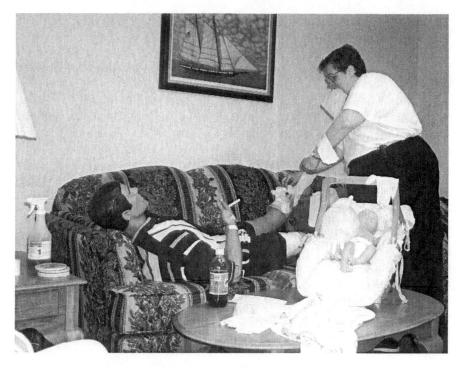

FIG. 10.2.   Improper infection control practices in the home.

The home environment is an essential component of the infection process that involves the patient as the host, agent of transmission, and reservoir; an infection cannot fester unless the host can live within the environment. The general environment is full of microorganisms that can be acutely or potentially harmful to humans. Figure 10.2 shows improper infection control in the home: the caregiver is using nonsterile techniques, the patient is smoking a cigarette, and the infant is located between the patient and caregiver, which could result in an injury to both the patient and the infant.

Hospitals and clinical settings are designed to control microorganisms in the environment; residential homes are not designed to serve as health-care settings. A suitable environment for home health care is one that has proper ventilation and enough exposure to the sun to prevent the growth of harmful fungi and bacteria. Few homes have that. Indeed, although homes have hand-washing facilities, few have appropriate conditions for disposal of environmental hazard materials—a potential source for infection. Home health care providers find their patients in homes that are conducive to infections, homes with excessive humidity, no running water, no refrigeration, and no heat or air conditioning. These conditions add additional tasks for the nurse, who must teach family members to use aseptic technique, good handwashing principles, and how to use or reuse equipment—tasks that are time consuming even for the most favorable home environment and usually not reimbursable.

Although it is necessary for home health care providers to incorporate effective infection control strategies in the home, the lack of medical equipment specifically designed for the home makes it difficult to provide an appropriate home environment that can reduce the potential of infection. Furthermore, the rationing of medical supplies caused by specific reimbursement patterns for home care makes the home environment even more difficult to control to prevent infections. The lack of professional staff such as home health aides, who have minimal training yet perform simple, necessary tasks, contributes to an increased risk of infection among homebound patients. For example, the home may have pets, children, extended-family members, or simply not enough space to house everyone—all of which are sources for potential infection. These factors negatively impact the overall care of an acutely ill patient who, due to reimbursement policy, was discharged in a barely subacute condition with invasive medical devices that are very difficult for the lay family caregiver to use.

As early as 1988, the importance of adapting new infection control standards specific to home health care was acknowledged (Rhinehart & Friedman, 1999). Recommendations for home health providers have been published on how to track and control postsurgical site infection, wound infections, and urinary tract infections, and infection control guidelines for surveillance for home care have been suggested (Valenti, 1994). When developed and disseminated, that information will assist home care providers in minimizing and controlling exposure to infections. It should be noted that these are guidelines rather than established mandatory regulations that monitor patient care and are tied to reimbursement. Thus, there is no impetus to spend time following guidelines, particularly when the workload is so heavy for home health care providers.

Patterns of Reimbursement

Jean found that Mrs. Tindell's HMO was closed on Saturday; the HMO did not authorize supplies or equipment and was not available on the weekend; the HMO did not authorize emergency services; the HMO physician would not authorize care because he was following criteria established by the insurance provider.

The health care industry and the government sought to decrease the cost of health care by early discharge of patients to the home. The pervasive use of technologically sophisticated equipment in the hospital setting has increased the cost of care, which makes hospitalization very expensive. By moving that equipment into the home and using lay caregivers, the health care industry has been able to reduce the total cost of care per patient. The use of technology to monitor patients in the home is considered a reasonable alternative to hospitalization by the industry and, indeed, has dramatically cut the cost of health care in the near term. These changes, however, have altered the image, scope, and practice of home health care nursing. Currently, society recognizes the value of home health care nursing as an essential, convenient alternative to hospitalization for managing chronic and acute health care problems. Reimbursement for these services, however, remains an issue.

As the demand for home health care services increased, private payers, HMOs, and the use of the federal reimbursement plans, Medicare and Medicaid, increased. Medicare is a federal program enacted by the United States Congress under title 18 of the Social Security Act of 1965 to provide reimbursement for health care for citizens 65 years of age and older and certain services such as dialysis for people of any age. Although the Medicare program offers coverage for home health care and hospice services in addition to inpatient hospital care, it requires that the patient be under direct supervision of a physician. The program offers fixed payment for services based on only one rate (Kravitz, Greenbold, & Rogers, 1992).

To avoid situations in which there is no Medicare reimbursement for services such as inpatient hospital care, health care providers quickly move the patients out of the hospital into their homes once they are stabilized. These changes have increased the level of acuteness of the conditions of patients in the home. This demands increased nursing skills by home health care providers. The pitfall for these services is that often the reimbursement is provided for a short period of time, covering only skilled nursing care and not nursing services for long-term or chronic conditions (Balinsky, 1985, 1994). The need for health care increases as a person ages; as the elderly population of the United States continues to increase, more and more home health services will be required, regardless of the reimbursement structures.

Medicaid, initiated in 1965, is a shared responsibility of both the local and federal governments to offer health care services to low-income citizens who are elderly, disabled, or children of low-income families. Medicaid covers many home health care services; however, Medicaid payments often are not sufficient to meet expenses for providing care. This leads many home health care agencies to not participate in the program (Dombi, 1994). Over 10,000 home health care agencies currently are certified for Medicare reimbursement. This certification is very important for many home health care agencies because it is a prerequisite for Medicaid certification (Spratt, Hawley, & Hoye, 1997). Although Medicare and Medicaid have largely contributed to the growth of the home health care industry, participation in these programs has not been free of financial problems.

Many private insurance companies provide home health services through HMOs. Most HMOs function on the principle that healthy individuals will counterbalance expenses incurred by less healthy people. To be profitable, more healthy than unhealthy people should be enrolled in the HMO. Because the growth of the elderly population is reflected in the number of elderly enrolled in an HMO and the elderly typically are increasingly in need of health care, the profits of many HMOs have plummeted. Therefore, a number of HMOs have dropped coverage for individuals with a chronic illness or patients who require longer nursing care services—typically elderly patients. Most HMOs limit the number of people they enroll; some HMOs have refused to provide coverage for Medicare populations ("Many Older Americans," 2000). If services are provided, they are physician controlled, diagnosis dependent, and often provide limited coverage (Kronick & Gilmer, 1999). Some HMOs provide financial incentives to physicians to keep the costs down by not ordering specific, often expensive, diagnostic tests, and by adhering to strict hospital admission policies and emergency room visits (Naylor, 1999). This is illustrated by Mrs. Dee's plight.

Recent advances in medicine have led to dramatic increases in the life expectancy among Americans. It is estimated that more than 60% of the general population in the United States will be over 65 in 2020 (Leon, Neuman, & Parente, 1997). As the population shifts from the young working class to a society of older Americans, the need will increase for managing chronic health problems of the elderly such as renal, heart, and respiratory illnesses. Prior to the use of technologically sophisticated equipment in the home, most elderly patients were hospitalized for prolonged periods of time. As technology changed inpatient care, so did the use of technology alter home care. Currently, most elderly patients receive care in their home via technologically sophisticated medical devices. This increases the demand for home health care services (Naylor, 1999).

Both patients and family members prefer that medical treatment be received in the home; such treatment has a number of benefits. The number of nosocomial infections—that is, infections acquired while in the hospital—is less among elderly patients discharged to their home for rehabilitation than among those who remain hospitalized (Lorenzen & Itkin, 1992). In addition, the patient and family members are more comfortable at home. The patients remain relatively independent by performing routine activities related to daily living (ADLs) and experience better outcomes at home (Ware, Kosinski, & Keller, 1996). Familiarity with the home environment provides an additional sense of comfort and security for the patient. The increasing use of home health care providers, technologically sophisticated devices, and family support at home are associated with positive patient outcomes (Rosenheimer, 1995). Indeed, elderly or acutely ill patients tend to have positive outcomes when family members are available to assist with their care or have the financial resources (insurance, private payment) available to pay for care. In general, the majority of the elderly population depends on the federal insurance programs of Medicare and Medicaid to provide nursing care or home care services.

Communication

Jean found that her patient, Mrs. Tindell, was not taught how to take care of her colostomy and her physician's on-call colleague (Dr. James) did not know her condition when returning Jean's call; the hospital discharge nurse did not obtain the needed oxygen equipment for Mr. Smith; and Mrs. Dee was not instructed about the impact of the diagnosis of Alzheimer's on a patient's condition.

Communication is the beginning of understanding. Health care professionals are trained as independent practitioners; they are not encouraged nor do they have time to develop interdisciplinary or multidisciplinary communication techniques on their own. For example, physicians and each of the allied health professional groups—which include nursing, pharmacy, and occupational and physical therapy—use different terms to refer to patient care needs. Each group has its own terminology when documenting patient care to such an extent that a glossary would be helpful to understand the care needs of patients. There are no formal information communication procedures that require the same nomenclature.

Currently, some of the Federal programs are mandating the use of the same medical diagnostic related group (DRG) terminology for reimbursement; however, services such as nursing and physical therapy are not reimbursed separately (Kravitz et al., 1992). Nursing fees for care such as administration of medication, monitoring of intravenous solutions, dressing changes, and the assessment of patients for complications resulting from their medications are not computer-entered; therefore, nursing actions or fees are not reimbursed. Often the rationale used has been that nursing and physical therapy are services that are integrated as part of the cost for a room or services that are provided as part of the total cost versus a defined cost. If all insurance providers, home health providers, and other health care providers were required to use the same language for reimbursement, there would be less confusion when providing and paying for patient care services. This would aid patients and family members in receiving needed care.

When the physician, nurse, and other hospital care providers communicate with each other and work together as a team, the patient has fewer complications and recovers quicker (Knaus, Draper, & Wagner, 1985). Such teamwork may be the exception rather than the rule, however. Often the physician discharges a patient to home care without adequate knowledge of the patient's ability to perform ADLs, relying on the inpatient nursing staff to recommend nursing care for the home. Family members typically are not taught how or when to provide care, as illustrated by Mrs. Kay's daughter.

Adverse events have occurred related to the improper use of medical devices such as the infusion pump used to give antibiotics to Mrs. Kay, respirators that breathe for a person, or other invasive technologies—improper because of misinformation or lack of information on how to use the device. The value of communication is evident in the improved performance and decrease of adverse events associated with team work and understanding information when military personnel are trained as teams to not only work together but also to manage their resources (Federal Aviation Administration, 1998). Surely, the health care industry can learn from examples and lessons learned in other domains such as the military and develop effective teamwork and communication to improve outcomes for home health care patients.

The Nursing Shortage

Jean was working overtime because the WECARE home health agency provided bonuses for staff who wanted to work more hours than the typical shift; the agency recently merged, resulting in demand for home health services for three times the number of patients. The nursing supervisor contacted several patients to notify them that they would have to wait an additional day for a nurse's visit.

Substantial changes in patient care requirements have created a critical shortage of qualified nurses. The American Organization of Nurse Executives (2002), American Nurses Association (1999), and the American Society for Health Care Human Resource Administration (ASHRA; 2002) reported the most critical nurse workforce priorities as flexible staffing for fluctuating patterns of patient care needs and organizational issues related to decreased reimbursement for nursing care. Previous national nurse shortage reports (ANA, 1999) addressed the issue of the aging nurse workforce and increased competition for qualified registered nurses. These reports indicate that future staffing needs include specialties such as community and home health, as well as medical, surgical, and critical care nurses.

Hospital and community health leaders as well as the public agree that nurses are the backbone of the health care system (ASHRA, 2002). Matching the type and supply of nurses to the demands for health care is essential. As the population ages, the need for home health care nurses exceeds the need for other nursing specialties by 50%, especially in rural areas (ANA, 1999). These rates are based on recruitment efforts; the national average time for successfully recruiting experienced home care nurses is 6 to 10 months.

National trends in the volume of cases for home care, that is, the number of cases per month, have changed markedly, demanding increased staffing to assure patient safety. For example, the average home care patient volume per agency was 10,000 patient visits per month, with predictions ranging from 17,000 to 21,000 patient care visits per month as home care agencies merge or are repurchased (Naylor, 1999). To meet staffing demands for home care nurses, home care agency administrators rely on travel nurses, temporary staff nurses, and personnel from temporary nurse agencies as well as targeted bonus options. They also rely on instituting training programs for nurses without home care experience to fill vacancies. Given the national average rate of 6 to 10 months to fill a home health care position, targeted action must be taken to ensure an adequate supply of competent and skilled nurses.

The national average age for nurses is 45 years; the national average age for home health nurses ranges between 50 to 55 years (ANA, 1999). Aging of the nursing workforce is at an all-time high. Nursing traditionally has been an appropriate profession for women; hence it has become dominated by women. Today, there are numerous other appropriate employment opportunities for women that lead students and mature women to choose careers other than nursing. Never before in the history of nursing has there been such a downward trend in the numbers of new graduates from nursing programs with respect to the number of nurses retiring. This means that as experienced nurses retire, fewer younger nurses or students are available, which perpetuates if not exacerbates the shortage of nurses.

The nursing shortage for home health nurses continues to be a major concern, particularly as the home health care industry grows (Naylor, 1999). Among the ways the nursing shortage affects consumers of home health services are the lack of certified nursing aides to provide basic nursing care needs such as bathing, wound care, and skin care, as well as the lack of registered nurses to provide health care to homebound patients. Specifically, registered nurses are needed to complete home health patient assessments such as physical exams or to monitor the effects of medications. Without enough home health nurses, patients can have severe medication reactions or display physical symptoms associated with illness and have more health complications from the lack of prevention. The shortage of nurses can be directly linked to adverse home health care patient outcomes such as the number of documented infections and patient falls as well as unmet patient needs. This is in addition to the number of patients unable to be seen by a home health nurse within 24 hours of when services have been requested (Irvine, Sidani, & Hall, 1998).

Technology and Medical Devices in the Home

Jean noted that the IV pump did not warn Mrs. Kay about an occlusion; an auto-mated air mattress remained deflated even after pushing the reset button; and a family member was not instructed about the use of oxygen for Mr. Smith.

The story of Mrs. Kay illustrates several issues related to the introduction of technologically sophisticated medical devices into the home. Driven by cost effectiveness and competition, health care services have moved from the hospital environment into patients' homes. Currently, home health care providers are faced with a plethora of medical equipment that was designed for hospital use and not for the home. Home care nurses must be able to work with any type of medical equipment ranging from an electronic thermometer to an ambulatory mechanical respiratory ventilator. The introduction of such equipment into the home has been convenient and cost effective; however, the risks associated with its use should not be overlooked (Kessler, Pape, & Sundwall, 1987).

The trends in health care have made intravenous infusion therapy—supplying a therapeutic medication in a person's vein using an infusion pump—a common practice in home health. Intravenous therapy in the home, however, is not free from potential complications. Such complications usually take place at the catheter insertion site or site where the needle is placed. Systemic infections are the most dangerous complications of IV therapy; frequently they are bloodstream infections that can be fatal. Proper insertion techniques and follow-up care such as cleaning the site, frequent dressing changes, and monitoring the infusion all play an important role in minimizing the risks of IV therapy-related infections. Homebound patients must be taught to keep their skin clean and maintain hygiene because microorganisms can migrate from the skin through an IV portal site to the bloodstream (Schaberg, Culver, & Gaynes, 1991).

Advances in technology have made it easier for home health care providers to carry out their assigned tasks. For example, the new approach for obtaining blood (transcutaneous phlebotomy) far exceeds the old approach in that it provides a way to obtain the least amount of blood in the safest manner while decreasing the risk of infection (Gingerich & Ondeck, 1996). Other examples of technology used in patient care include the use of satellite monitoring of a patient's heart rate, blood sugar, or pulse rate. In today's world, communication technology such as e-mails, the Internet, telemedicine, and satellite cell phones has been utilized to monitor multiple home health patients. Nonetheless, a great deal of work has yet to be done to invent medical equipment that is reliable, user friendly, and safe for the home care provider. Home health care equipment must be designed so that family members can use it without being fearful of error. Given the introduction of technologically sophisticated medical devices in home care, it is important that a means for quality assessment of their use be put in place to assure nurses, nursing assistants, and other staff of safe operation of such devices, together with fail-safe mechanical engineering of the devices to assure patient safety in the home (Gallivan, 1997).

A DAY IN THE LIFE

The stories of Mrs. Tindell, Mr. Smith, Mrs. Kay, and Mr. Dee that occur in a day in the life of Mrs. Jean Lowe may appear unreal or overly drastic; however, they are real—snapshots of the reality of home care nursing. The current trends in health care delivery that promote short hospital stays to reduce costs, merge health care organizations, and restrict information, set the stage for days in which providing home care is frustrating, fragmented, and wrought with multiple opportunities for adverse events. Although Jean was well educated and an experienced nurse, it was necessary for her to continuously compensate for problems resulting from lack of communication among health care personnel and insurance providers.

Jean had to troubleshoot many factors associated with the planning and implementation of patient care, often spending an inordinate amount of time coordinating efforts to obtain home equipment and facilitating communication between and among various health care providers, insurance companies, and paramedical groups. Jean had minimal information about the patients—only their name, diagnosis, and discharge date—prior to entering the home, yet she was responsible and accountable for providing comprehensive nursing care. Jean was familiar with the home environment; she had provided nursing care in the home as a home health aide for more than 3 years and she had the knowledge of a baccalaureate education. Although her intentions were to complete care for all her assigned patients, she was constantly delayed by spending more time per patient than she intended trying to deal with factors from dysfunctional health care services.

Jean was a victim of a complex assortment of health care services that lacks the infrastructure necessary to provide continuity of care for patients from the time they are hospitalized until they have recovered at home or have an established health care regimen for a chronic condition. Sooner or later, Jean could be held accountable and possibly sued because she was not able to reach a patient's home to provide care in a timely fashion. Family members of home health patients tend to be so distressed by the demands and frustrations of trying to provide adequate care that by the time a nurse reaches them, they are grateful for someone to help, so litigation cases against nurses in home health nursing remain low. What is most upsetting in the stories of Mrs. Tindell, Mr. Smith, Mrs. Kay, and Mr. Dee is the fact that Jean, a competent and caring home health nurse, will become burned out and eventually change to another type of nursing specialty or leave.

Of the 2.4 million nurses available to work in the United States, more than half of them change careers, enter new careers, or elect not to work (ANA, 1999). This is a sad commentary for a nation whose population is aging and whose need for home health care services is expanding. Jean has been a nurse for only 1 year; eventually she will become frustrated from her daily work as she encounters more and more problems with the health services. She may not encourage—indeed may even discourage—others who are considering entering the nurse workforce.

Nurses are aware of all aspects of health care because they are responsible for the 24-hour monitoring of patient care; no other health care professional is involved in solving the myriad of problems related to 24-hour care. Others are aware only of their aspect of health care and as such are not affected by the fragmentation of routine patient care activities. All too often, home care nurses leave the profession or change careers within nursing because they feel helpless in an archaic system. Jean continued working for the home health care agency immersed in the daily frustration of working among factors that thwart her best efforts to provide home health care—factors that contribute to, if not induce, error.

REFERENCES

American Nurses Association. (1999). *Report about the nursing shortage: What are the options.* Washington, DC: Author.

American Organization of Nurse Executives. (2002, January 30). *New Survey Provides Insight into Nursing Field.* Washington, DC: Author.

American Society for Health Care Human Resource Administration. (2002). *Building a framework for workforce: Solution.* Chicago, IL: Author.

Association of Practitioners in Infection Control. (1999). *Guidelines for infection control in home health settings.* Washington, DC: Author.

Balinsky, W. (Ed.). (1994). *Home care: Current problems and future solutions.* San Francisco: Jossey-Bass.

Balinsky, W. (1985). Home care: Current trends and future prospects. *New York Business Group on Health Discussion Papers, 22*(1), 40–45.

Chassin, M., & Gavin, R. (1998). The urgent need to improve health care quality. *Journal of the American Medical Association, 280*(11), 1000–1005.

Chusid, J. (1987). Standards needed to improve home care quality. *American Nurse, 19*(5), 10, 18.

Dombi, W. (1994, May 10–20). Legal issues in home care. *Caring, 13*(5), 12–16, 18–20.

Federal Aviation Administration. (1998). The human factors guide for aviation maintenance and inspection (version 3) and FAA human factors in aviation maintenance and inspection Internet website. http://hfskyway.faa.gov.

Gallivan, M. (1997). *Global medical technology update: The challenges facing U.S. industry and policy makers.* Washington, DC: Health Manufacturers Association.

Gingerich, B., & Ondeck, D. (Eds.). (1996). *Home health redesign: A proactive approach to managed care.* Gaithersburg, MD: Aspen.

Haddad, A., & Kapp, M. (Eds.). (1991). *Ethical and legal issues in home health care.* Norwalk, CT: Appleton & Lange.

Hellinghausen, M. A. (1999, January 14). Burdens of care: Helping home caregivers to be mindful of their own health. Retrieved from www.nurseweek.com/features/99-/care.html

Institute of Medicine. (1999). *To err is human: Building a safer health system.* Washington, DC: National Academy Press.

Irvine, D., Sidani, S., & Hall, L. M. (1998). Linking outcomes to nurse's roles in healthcare. *Nursing Economics, 16*(21), 58–64.

Joel, L. (1989). Professionalizing the nursing home. *American Nurse, 21*(4), 7.

Kessler, D. A., Pape, S. M., & Sundwall, D. (1987). The federal regulation of medical devices. *New England Journal of Medicine, 317,* 357–366.

Knaus, W., Draper, E., & Wagner, D. (1985). APACHE II: A severity for disease classification system. *Critical Care Medicine, 13,* 818–829.

Kravitz, R., Greenbold, S., & Rogers W. (1992). Differences in the mix of patients among medical specialties and systems of care. Results from the medical outcomes study. *Journal of the American Medical Association, 267,* 1617–1623.

Kronick, R., & Gilmer, T. (1999). Explaining the decline in health insurance coverage: 1979–1995. *Health Affairs, 18*(2), 30–47.

Leon, J., Neuman, P., & Parente, S. (1997). *Understanding the growth in Medicare home health expenditures.* Bethesda, MD: Project Hope Center for Health Affairs.

Many older Americans in search of alternate health coverage. (2000, August 2). *The Baltimore Sun,* p. 32.

Lorenzen, A. N., & Itkin, D. J. (1992). Surveillance of infection in home care. *American Journal of Infection Control, 20*(6), 326–329.

Naylor, M. (1999). Comprehensive home care after hospitalization of elderly patients. *Journal of the American Medical Association, 282*(29), 11–29.

Rhinehart, E., & Friedman, M. (Eds.). (1999). *Infection control in home care.* Gaithersburg, MD: Association of Practitioners in Infection Control.

Rosenheimer, L. (1995). Establishing a surveillance system for infection acquired in home care. *Home Nurse, 13*(3), 20–26.

Schaberg, D. R., Culver, D. H., & Gaynes, R. P. (1991). Major trends in the microbial etiology of nosocomial infection. *American Journal of Medicine, 91,* 72s–75s.

Spratt, J., Hawley, R., & Hoye, R. (Eds.). (1997). *Home health care: Principles and practice.* Delray Beach, FL: GR/St. Lucie Press.

Thomas, E. J., Studdert, D. M., & Newhouse, J. (1999). Costs of medical injuries in Utah and Colorado. *Inquiry, 3,* 255–264.

Valenti, W. M. (1994). Infection control, human immunodeficiency virus, and home health care: 1. Infection risks to the patient. *American Journal of Infection Control, 22,* 370–372.

Ware, J., Kosinski, M., & Keller, S. D. (1996). A 12-item short-form health survey: Construction of scales and preliminary tests of reliability and validity. *Medical Care, 34*(3), 220–233.

11

Aging, Cognition, and Patient Errors in Following Medical Instructions

Denise C. Park
The University of Illinois

Ian Skurnik
The University of Toronto

SENIOR CITIZENS, GEORGE AND NANCY MULLEN

George and Nancy Mullen are ages 82 and 78, respectively, and have been married for 56 years. George is a retired autoworker and has good medical care benefits. After George retired at age 62, he and Nancy enjoyed a period of good health and relative financial ease. They owned two modest homes: a lake cottage in northern Michigan and a bungalow in Florida. They traveled between the two homes, living in each for 6 months a year. Some of their aging brothers and sisters owned homes in the same two areas and they enjoyed a happy and social retirement.

In the past few years, however, the Mullens, who have been quite independent, have faced significant challenges due to failing health. George, a life-long smoker, developed emphysema. Even though he stopped smoking, the emphysema quickly became severe enough to limit his mobility—sometimes taking just 4 or 5 steps made him feel as if he were suffocating and required him to rest before continuing. He needed additional oxygen, from portable tanks, on a regular basis to breathe. At first, this condition frustrated George and he would occasionally sneak a cigarette. This was extraordinarily risky because in addition to accelerating his emphysema, the act of smoking could ignite the oxygen tanks that were at his side constantly. Recently, George became morose about his condition and was diagnosed with depression by his family physician. In an effort to alleviate his depression, Zoloft was prescribed for him. When this did not work, an MAO inhibitor was prescribed. The MAO inhibitor was effective in treating his depression, but brought on a host of side effects and involved dietary restrictions such as no dairy products.

Nancy Mullen, George's wife, had suffered for some time from hypertension and mild diabetes; recently she developed macular degeneration. With this condition, her eyesight deteriorated steadily. She was beginning to have trouble reading books, newspapers, and prescription labels, as well as paying bills and shopping. Nancy takes two hypertension medications and three medications for her diabetes daily, in addition to an assortment of vitamin and mineral supplements. Nancy and George frequently take over-the-counter (OTC) preparations for their health based on information from friends, television shows, newspapers, and magazines. Unfortunately, some of the OTC products have worked against their regular medical care by interacting with prescription drugs to create their own side effects, as well as to compromise the effectiveness of the prescription medications.

One of the Mullen's children, Pamela Barber, lives about 30 miles away and tries to help her parents with their medical needs. She already is busy at a demanding professional position as a human resource manager for a large company, as well as being a single mother of two teenagers. She barely manages to meet the demands of her job and the needs of her children; she feels guilty that she does not always have time to attend to the steadily increasing health care needs of her parents. In her efforts to provide what care she can, Pamela frequently is puzzled by her parents' explanations about their health status and doctors' visits. She is concerned that her parents do not take their medications correctly or follow the instructions of the health care providers. Pamela has come to believe that inadvertent errors in self-care by her parents create additional medical problems. She also is concerned that in addition to making errors in taking medications because they fail to understand or follow physician instructions, her parents may come to harm because of the OTC herbs and minerals they are taking. She believes her parents remember only fragments of what they read or hear in the media about these products, which leads to confusion about what is effective.

Pamela began to talk directly with her parents' physicians to better understand their diagnoses and prognoses. She was not surprised to learn that sometimes the physicians need to spend extra time with her parents to explain treatments and conditions. Given the garbled information her parents tell her they received from their physicians, Pamela was astonished that the physicians believed her parents understood quite well what they were told. For example, the physician had spent considerable time explaining to Nancy Mullen that an herbal treatment she was taking for her diabetes is ineffective and could even be dangerous. The physician told Pamela that he felt her mother understood that she should not take the herb. Later, Nancy told Pamela that she believed this herbal remedy would have a beneficial effect on her diabetes. Pamela was frustrated that her parents seem to consistently misunderstand information and translate the misunderstanding into dangerous medical behaviors.

In addition to her parents' health problems, Pamela was recently diagnosed with rheumatoid arthritis, a systemic, progressive condition that results in considerable fatigue and requires her to take seven different medications to treat inflammation, pain, and autoimmune activity. Her prognosis is good if she carefully adheres to her medication schedule and does not become overly fatigued; however, this regimen is proving more difficult than she anticipated. Pamela recognizes that because of her extremely busy schedule, she has difficulty taking her medications at the right times of day, so although she understands what she needs to do with the medications, Pamela misses many doses. Pamela's medical errors are playing a role in her own debilitated health.

COGNITIVE CHANGES
AND SELF-CARE ERROR

The scenario just described has two important themes. First, as George and Nancy Mullen advance into their 80s, they are experiencing normal age-related declines in cognitive function at the same time that their medical problems and medical regimens become increasingly complex. As a result of this combination, problems in comprehension and memory are manifest in errors in self-administered medication. Second, Pamela, a middle-aged adult, is having trouble remembering to take her medications correctly, despite the fact that her cognitive function is at a high level, because she is so stressed by the many demands on her. Pamela's situation underscores the point that not all patient-based medical errors occur in older adults, and not all errors are due to misunderstanding. Contextual factors that demand the attention of individuals to the extent that they cannot remember to attend to their medical needs can play an important role in medical errors, particularly in busy, middle-aged adults.

George and Nancy Mullen can decrease the errors due to their aging cognitive abilities by using environmental cues, reminders, and other cognitive supports. Pamela, in contrast, can accommodate the effect of stress on her cognitive functioning by structuring factors in her environment so they do not interfere with her ability to care for her health problems. This family's ability to engage in medical care and decrease the likelihood of possible medical errors depends on an interaction of their cognitive systems and their health behaviors, all within the context in which their medical care is imbedded—that of the media, work, and social systems such as family.

Age-Related Changes in Cognition and Memory

What happens to people's cognitive systems as they age? Can the declines in cognitive function that occur in late adulthood be responsible for medical errors? It is common for people to fear that their memory will decline as they age. The debilitating affects of Alzheimer's disease are the extreme, but not the only age-related impairment of cognitive functioning. It is important to recognize that even healthy adults age 65 and older experience some changes in their cognitive functioning (for recent reviews, see Craik & Jennings, 1992; Park, 2000).

One aspect of cognitive functioning that changes with age is the speed of cognitive processing or the speed with which a person can process information—for example, how rapidly one can perform mental operations, such as comparing two strings of digits to be the same or different. With age, mental operations are slowed, which, depending on the degree of slowness, can have a profound effect on the ability to comprehend and remember information (Salthouse, 1996). Thus, one reason for the Mullens' difficulties in implementing their doctors' instructions may be that they are not able to absorb very much of the information presented to them about their health problems. The physician often tells them about their health problems at a rapid rate with little if any time to ask for elaboration or questions. Cognitive processing, indeed cognitive functioning, involves several types of memory; however, memory deficits in older adults are not universal for all types of memory situations.

Older adults are nearly as adept as younger adults in recalling that they have heard a piece of information before (often called old–new recognition memory); yet they are noticeably poorer than younger adults in remembering the context in which they heard the information (source memory), or in reorganizing and manipulating information in their heads (working memory). The problems older adults experience can be different for short-term memory (memory of recent occurrences or information) and for long-term memory. In other words, aging is not necessarily accompanied by a general, across-the-board decline in all cognitive abilities. Instead, a particular pattern of age-related declines is apparent.

Cognitive processing declines are greatest for those tasks that require fast mental processing or extensive cognitive effort, as in making a quick decision that involves a number of considerations such as deciding which of several vacations to take before the expiration of a special price. Cognitive declines in older adults are small or nonexistent when the tasks rely on knowledge.

For working memory, the effects of aging are not unique to people over 65. Those effects can be closely mimicked in younger adults by putting them in situations of high distraction, time pressure, and fatigue. For example, if younger adults are required to study words while at the same time monitoring whether a stream of digits is odd or even, their performance on studying words will be similar to that of older adults who do not monitor the digits (Craik & Jennings, 1992; Park, 2000). The task of digit monitoring decreases the working memory capacity in the younger adults so that it approximates the age-compromised working memory of older adults.

Another limitation George and Nancy face is a decrease in working memory capacity. That decrease likely contributes to their making errors in following treatment regimens. Consider that George and Nancy and Pamela Barber need to be able to understand a good deal of new information when they visit their health care providers. That information can consist of new medical terms and names, presented in the complex ways typical of medical professionals, as well as new treatment regimens. Not only do they have to understand all of this information, they have to integrate it into a treatment plan compatible with their everyday lives outside the physician's office. This is a challenge because George and Nancy and their daughter, Pamela, like everyone else, are distracted by other concerns; because of cognitive declines and stress, respectively, they may not be able to resist such distractions.

All aspects of memory involved in receiving instructions from a health care provider—comprehending new information, storing it effectively in memory, and retrieving that information later—depend to some degree on working memory. The age-related pattern of decline in cognitive processing and working memory, as well as impaired long-term memory, all contribute to the difficulties that George and Nancy have in appropriately following their doctor's instructions. Working memory particularly is important in following instructions because it involves the ability to manipulate, code, and retrieve information. To experience the role of working memory in mental tasks, continue to read this paragraph, while at the same time counting backwards by twos from 100. Either reading or counting backwards is easy enough alone; however, doing both tasks simultaneously demands more mental resources than a person can smoothly allocate (Baddeley, 1994). To compensate for the difficulty of both reading and counting at the same time, avoid making mistakes, and learn from reading, it is necessary to perform the tasks slowly.

The age-related changes in cognitive function do not occur when a person reaches 60 years of age; rather, beginning as early as in one's 20s, there is a slow, gradual decline in both speed of processing and working memory that becomes quite pronounced as a person ages. Such decreases in speed of processing and working memory capacity limit memory for long-term information (Park et al., 1996; Park et al., 2002), comprehension of new information, as well as reasoning, problem solving, and decision making (Craik, Anderson, Kerr, & Li, 1995; Light, 1991). It is not generally well recognized that these declines begin in young adulthood and that the declines in speed of processing, working memory, and long-term memory are gradual, continuous, and linear across the lifespan

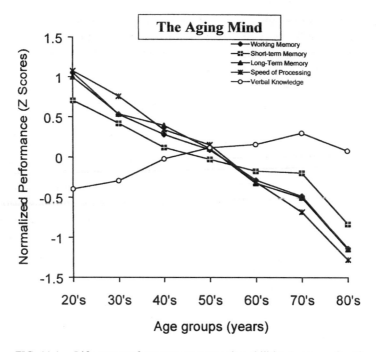

FIG. 11.1.   Life-span performance on processing abilities (a composite of speed of processing, working memory, short-term memory, and long-term memory) and verbal knowledge. Higher scores represent better performance. (Adapted from Park et al., 2002. Copyright © 2002 by the American Psychological Association. Adapted by permission.)

(Baltes & Lindenberger, 1997; Park et al., 1996; Park et al., 2002). The gentle downward slope of the decline in cognitive function that begins in a person's 20s reaches a considerable decline when people reach their 80s. This is in contrast to a common belief that people's cognitive abilities function at a constant level, plateau, and decline in a cliff-like manner when they reach the later adulthood of ages 60 or 70 years.

The lifespan relationships between aging and cognition are represented in Fig. 11.1 (adapted from Park et al., 2002). Those relationships indicate that as a person ages, there are regular, linear declines in cognitive processing, working memory, and long-term memory. Such changes occur at the same time a person's vocabulary, which often is considered as representing a person's world knowledge, remains intact or actually grows. Thus, at the same time continuous declines in cognitive processes occur, aging adults are gaining knowledge and expertise that are stored in memory to be drawn upon as new experiences and information are encountered.

Examination of the lines in Fig. 11.1 for the younger ages finds that the cognitive processing of young adults is very quick to take in new information; however, young adults have considerably less knowledge and experience than older adults. The decreases evidenced in Fig. 11.1 become particularly important for errors in self-care in late-mid to late adulthood. In those years, slowed cognitive processing and decreases in working memory and long-term memory can have a significant impact on how unfamiliar medical information, instructions, and equipment are understood. These are some of the factors that contribute to the problems the George and Nancy are having managing their health. Let us return to the Mullens and their daughter for an update on their situation.

Because of concern about Nancy Mullen's diabetes affecting her eyesight and her macular degeneration she, accompanied by her husband, went to a major medical center for a complete vision workup. Nancy spent 5 hours at the medical center, during which she encountered eight different health care professionals—residents, physicians, and assistants—who conducted various tests in an assortment of contexts that left her exhausted. Finally, Nancy met with her primary ophthalmologist, Dr. Michaels.

Dr. Michaels integrated the findings from the various tests and presented her situation to Nancy. He told her that she has a serious condition: a type of macular degeneration that is not treatable because of the diffuse nature of the blood vessel damage in her retina. Her focal vision is rapidly being obliterated and shortly she will have only peripheral vision. Although she had not realized the extent of changes in her vision, Dr. Michaels told Nancy her vision has become so poor that she meets the criteria to be declared legally blind. He informed her of a number of available assistive devices that will be of tremendous help to her in maximizing the use of her peripheral vision so she can maintain her daily routines. Additionally, Dr. Michaels told her that the local association for the blind can provide her with additional information and assistance and provide her with recorded books and magazines for the blind. He also told Nancy that certain financial and tax advantages accrue to individuals declared to be legally blind; however, she must enroll for this and other services in person because there are papers and forms to be completed. At the conclusion of the visit, Nancy and George were given an opportunity to ask questions, but they had none; they were given no written materials to take home and study about Nancy's condition or contact information for the services Dr. Michaels described.

After her day at the medical center and meeting with Dr. Michaels, George and Nancy returned home and Nancy talked with their daughter about the physician's report. Nancy was unable to tell Pamela the nature of the vision problem that the various tests indicated she has or the treatment Dr. Michaels proposed for it. She appeared uncertain about the seriousness of her condition and its prognosis. This frustrated Pamela because all that was clear from talking with her mother was that her mother has some type of retinal problem that apparently is serious and requires some type of treatment. Her father, George, was unable to add any information to what his wife reported.

Nancy very much wanted Pamela to call Dr. Michaels to learn about her condition. Pamela made the call and told Dr. Michaels how the information her mother provided about her vision problem from her meeting with him was sparse and vague. He was astonished to learn that Nancy had so little understanding of what they had discussed. Without consulting his records, Dr. Michaels recalled Nancy Mullen and her condition in detail and indicated that he discussed her treatment with her and her husband for over 30 minutes. He then reviewed with Pamela everything he discussed with her mother and remarked several times that Nancy seemed to understand every word that he said, so he was surprised that she could not relate to her daughter at least some of what they discussed about her condition. He particularly commented on how astute and engaged she appeared in his office.

Comprehension of a Medical Condition.   Both young and older adults must go through a number of cognitive steps to adequately receive information about treatment for a diagnosed medical condition (Park, 1992). For the Mullens, something clearly went awry in the transfer of information from physician to patient, which resulted in very little information transferred from patient to daughter. In this first step of securing effective medical treatment, Nancy Mullen did not adequately understand her health problem from the information presented to her. As shown in Fig. 11.1, working memory and speed of cognitive processing decrease with age, which places older adults at risk of having difficulty comprehending medical interactions. This was exacerbated for Nancy Mullen by an exhausting day of tests, meetings, waiting, and more meetings, in addition to the unfamiliar environments of the medical center—conditions that would adversely affect anyone.

Because of cognitive declines that occur as a natural part of aging, older adults have more difficulty understanding a number of aspects of medical care than younger adults (Park & Hall-Gutchess, 2000). For example, older adults do not understand straightforward medication regimens presented in a simulated medical environment as well as younger adults (Morrell, Park, & Poon, 1989). This occurs regardless of the format in which the information is presented, even if it appears in simple pictures with minimal text in pamphlets designed by hospitals for actual patients. This lack of understanding is not unique to medical information; older adults do not comprehend information about living wills and advanced directives as well as younger adults (Zwahr, Park, Eaton, & Larson, 1997). Both hospital and nursing home administrators have reported their biggest concern about the Patient Self-Determination Act implemented by Congress, that directs their facilities to provide opportunities for the older patients to create living wills and advanced directives, is having them understand the information (Park, Eaton, Larson, & Palmer, 1994).

With respect to their own health care, older compared to younger adults spend less time on medical decisions and are less sophisticated in considering information about medical decisions for potentially life-threatening conditions, such as breast cancer (Meyer, Russo, & Talbot, 1995), or for more common conditions, such as whether to take estrogen replacement therapy (Zwahr, Park, & Shifren, 1999). For example, when making decisions about estrogen replacement therapy after reading a detailed pamphlet, older women compared to younger women on average considered fewer options, made fewer comparative judgments among choices, and had an overall lower quality of reasons for decisions they made. The relatively impoverished judgments and lack of consideration of options by older compared to younger women were attributed to the lowered speed of cognitive processing and compromised working memory— the mechanisms noted in Fig. 11.1. Education also plays an important and direct role in the options that older women understood; the more education, the more the women understood their options.

As cognitive resources decline, older more than younger adults are at a disadvantage when they must assimilate entirely novel information about a condition in an unfamiliar environment (Park, 1994). Thus, one major factor contributing to inappropriate patient decisions leading to error in self-care and negative treatment outcomes is the lack of comprehension of medical information that occurs at the time a physician talks with and instructs older patients. Offering older adults various environmental supports can enhance their comprehension and decision-making capabilities and reduce the likelihood of error in self-care. Among those supports are written information to take home, opportunities to phone and ask questions of a physician's assistant, and opportunities to obtain additional information on the use of medical devices and medications from training sessions and clinics, as well as videotapes, books, organizational newsletters, and web-sites. Despite the areas of cognitive decline associated with normal aging, older adults have cognitive strengths.

COGNITIVE STRENGTHS OF OLDER ADULTS

Despite the older women's relatively inappropriate reasoning for their decisions regarding estrogen replacement therapy, their ultimate decisions were the same as younger women; only the basis for the decision differed (Zwahr et al., 1999). Older adults, if for no other reason than they have lived longer than younger adults, have had more medical interactions on average, so in some ways they are expert consumers and users of health care (Park, 1999). In addition, their verbal skills are equal or superior to those of young adults (Park et al., 1996), which should enable older adults to make considerable use of supplementary materials, given enough time to review them. Nancy Mullen was given information verbally about her new condition that, to be assimilated, required considerable working memory and speed of cognitive processing. George and Nancy might better have understood details about Nancy's condition if they had been given written information to take home where they could review the new material without the need for speedy cognitive processing and immediately accessible memory.

Some of the difficulty George and Nancy experienced understanding what Dr. Michaels told them about Nancy's condition is that older adults do not learn new information about a familiar disease such as breast cancer and an unfamiliar disease such as acromegaly as readily as younger adults (Brown & Park, in press). For George and Nancy, the familiar disease was Nancy's diabetes-related vision problems. An explanation for this counterintuitive finding may be that it is difficult for older adults to learn information inconsistent with or disconfirming what they already believe. Because Nancy Mullen had macular degeneration for some time and believed she knew the nature of that condition, it may have been particularly difficult for her to learn the new information about how serious that medical condition had become.

Aging and Medication Adherence

Given the declining cognitive capabilities associated with normal aging, it has been widely believed that older adults are at substantially greater risk of nonadherence to medical regimens than younger adults. There is no question that older adults compared with younger adults are the larger consumers of medical care and take more medications, with an estimate of 2.9 prescriptions per older adult (Kiernan & Isaacs, 1981). Self-reported rates of nonadherence to medication regimens for older adults are quite high (Bergman & Wilhom, 1981; Botelho & Dudrak, 1992); however, information on medication adherence obtained without relying on self-reports presents a very different picture than the conventional wisdom.

Older adults compared with younger adults often are *more* adherent to regimens and make fewer errors in taking medications (Green, Mullen, & Stainbrook, 1986; Richardson, Simons-Morton, & Annegers, 1993). The oldest category of adults, those aged 75+, and middle-aged individuals, ages 45 to 64, tend to make the most adherence errors, with young-old adults, aged 65 to 74, making the fewest errors (Morrell, Park, Kidder, & Martin, 1997; Park, Morrell,

Frieske, & Kincaid, 1992). Thus, it appears that older adults adhere to medication regimens quite well until very late adulthood, although adherence rates differ substantially among adults aged 60 to 90.

Various reasons have been suggested for why seniors aged roughly 65 to 75 make relatively few medication errors despite the age-related cognitive declines they are experiencing. A general explanation can be that the cognitive functioning of young-old adults is sufficient for them to be highly adherent to medication regimens until very late adulthood, when that functioning becomes compromised and becomes a factor in nonadherence. This is a reason why the oldest-old make the most adherence errors, and young-old the least. Given that adults in the 60 to 75 year range experience substantial cognitive decline as illustrated in Fig. 11.1, the trend in adherence for adults 65 to 75 years old suggests that noncognitive factors, as well as cognitive factors, play an important role in self-administered medication errors. (For further reading on medication adherence, see Park & Jones, 1996; Park & Kidder, 1996; Park & Mayhorn, 1996)

CONTEXTUAL FACTORS, AGING, AND COMPREHENSION

Based on what is known about the relative contributions of medical status, cognitive status, psychological variables, and social context in explaining self-care medication errors, George and Nancy Mullen and their middle-aged daughter Pamela are all at high risk of committing errors through nonadherence to medication regimens, but for different reasons. George and Nancy are both in late adulthood, when declining cognitive functioning plays an increasing role in nonadherence (Park et al., 1992). For their 45-year-old daughter Pamela, the biggest risk factor for nonadherence is a self-reported busy lifestyle (Park et al., 1999). Adults, typically middle-aged, who report having busy, unpredictable lifestyles, seem to be at greatest risk of nonadherence. Thus, Pamela Barber, who is not exhibiting significant cognitive decline, is at risk for medical nonadherence because she is a single parent with a demanding job who is also trying to help her aged parents. Younger adults have the cognitive resources to manage medications, but often feel sufficient pressure from the environment that they are unable to remember to take their medications accurately. Reminding devices such as beeping wristwatches can be effective devices in improving medication adherence errors for busy people (Park, Shifren, & Morrell, 1998).

Belief in False Information

Pamela Barber also was concerned that her parents misconstrued warnings that their physicians gave them about self-care and medications; for example, that herbal supplements are ineffective in treating Nancy Mullen's diabetes. Their physicians told Nancy and George that information they may obtain that states that herbal supplements would help is not true; however, they seemed to believe it was. This flip-flop in beliefs is part of a well-documented memory distortion called the *illusion of truth,* which occurs when sheer repetition of statements increases the perceived truth (Begg, Anas, & Farinacci, 1992; Gilbert, Krull, & Malone, 1990; Hasher, Goldstein, & Toppino, 1977). It seems to occur when people realize they have heard a piece of information before, but cannot remember the source—that is, who said it, where they heard it, or the context in which it was presented. This illusion is that if people believe they have heard information before, it probably is true. That strategy might be accurate most of the time, but it can lead to serious mistakes when the information was not true. That is, the illusion of truth is dangerous because it can make false information seem true and create serious errors in the medical realm.

The illusion of truth is a robust effect to which both older and younger adults are susceptible. Because of a particular pattern of age-related declines in memory performance, older adults are at greater risk for mistakenly remembering false information as true. Specifically, barring clinical memory disorders such as Alzheimer's disease, older adults have nearly the same ability as younger adults to discriminate previously presented information from information that they have never seen (Spencer & Raz, 1995). This ability often is referred to as a capacity to experience a vague feeling of familiarity, similar to the feeling that underlies a déjà vu experience or a tip-of-the-tongue state (Jacoby & Dallas, 1981; Mandler, 1980).

Older adults tend to have deficits in remembering the source of information or the clear contextual details that would help identify the context in which the information was acquired (Johnson, DeLeonardis, Hashtroudi, & Ferguson, 1995). A prototypic example of this type of memory might be when an older adult remembers that someone told them there would be thunderstorms next week, but cannot remember who it was. This pattern of intact and impaired memory performance—preserved feelings of familiarity but impaired source memory—indicates that older adults are increasingly susceptible to the illusion of truth effect (Mutter, Lindsey, & Pliske, 1995).

Older adults show a stronger illusion of truth effect than do younger adults (Law, Hawkins, & Craik, 1998; Mutter et al., 1995). They are vulnerable to a paradoxical rebound effect in which repeated warnings that information is false backfires and the information subsequently is likely to be considered true. Repeated warnings that a statement is false—for example, "It's not true that shark cartilage alleviates arthritis"—intuitively should make it easier to remember than a single warning. Such repeated warnings do help both younger and older adults remember the warning accurately in the short term, thus avoiding the illusion of truth. After 3 days, however, if older adults were told repeatedly that the statement is false, rather than if they were told just once, they are more likely than younger adults to think that shark cartilage benefits arthritis (Skurnik, Park, & Schwarz, 2000). Thus, in the longer term, the initial beneficial effect of repeated warnings backfires for older adults and the repeated false information is considered as being true; the advantage of repetition persists in younger adults and they accurately remember the statement as false.

Just as Pamela Barber observed, the conscientious physician repeatedly told the Mullens not to believe that the herbal supplement helped Nancy Mullen's diabetes. They were able to remember this when they were still in the physician's office; however, after some time had passed, the repeated information was still familiar, but details about the exact circumstance in which it had been learned were starting to fade. The paradoxical consequence is that over time false information seemed true (the herbal supplement was good for the diabetes)—not in spite of, but *because of* repeated warnings about it being false. In addition, characteristics of obtaining health care, as illustrated by Nancy's fatigue and stress of a day at a medical center, can only add to the risk of memory distortions such as the illusion of truth for both younger and older adults, which can lead to subsequent medical errors.

Environmental Supports to Minimize Medical Errors

The key to increasing source memory for information, and therefore to minimizing the illusion of truth effect, is to provide contextual support, such as reading materials for reference or to use to cue specific memories. Often environmental support can compensate for the negative effects of cognitive aging, and the more support the better for contextual memory tasks. When older adults have materials that support memory at both encoding (the time they first learn information) and retrieval (the time they recall the information), they can often perform nearly as well as younger adults (Craik, Byrd, & Swanson, 1987; Craik & Jennings, 1992). Younger adults are not immune to paradoxical memory illusions; distraction and time pressure often produce the same pattern of memory distortions that are evident in older adults (Jacoby, 1999). Pamela Barber was surprised to learn of her parents' belief in false information, but her life circumstances may make her just as vulnerable to the effect as George and Nancy.

Contextual cues and supporting materials would help the Mullens with a number of source memory tasks that they might face, such as the illusion of truth effect. Because George is unemotional and depressed in medical settings, Nancy is the primary means of communication with the health care professionals. She must remember his symptoms as well as her own so she can report them to the doctors; she also must remember each of their treatment plans so she can implement them. The risk of confusing the details of one person's plan with that of another without support of written material seems great for Nancy and George.

The environmental support provided by medication organizers that are divided into compartments for pills can decrease errors in complying with a medication regimen. It is essential, however, that the organizers be filled correctly, because once the pills and tablets are put in an organizer, the name and other information about the medication are not associated with the specific medication. Patients are particularly prone to load medication organizers incorrectly if they have only seven large compartments, one for each day of the week (Park, Morrell, Frieske, Blackburn, & Birchmore, 1992). In such organizers, both the information about the identity of the medication and the instructions for taking it are on the bottles, which then are separate from the medication. Thus, a memory aid for minimizing errors—the organizer—could contribute to errors, so it is important to be vigilant and not assume that an OTC device designed to reduce medical errors will not actually contribute to error. Medication organizers that have four slots for each of the seven days of the week are more likely to be loaded correctly and facilitate adherence in the very old (Park et al., 1992).

A dimension of medication errors that has not received much attention is the prospect that each member of a couple may act as an environmental support or memory aide for the other. In some cases, elderly individuals living alone made more medication errors than elderly people who lived with a spouse, significant other, or sibling. This likely is due to the lack of another individual to help organize a medication regimen and serve as a reminder to take the medications (Park et al., 1992; Schwartz, Wand, Zeitz, & Goss, 1962). Similarly, spousal support following a coronary episode plays an important role in regimen adherence (Doherty, Schrott, Metcalf, & Iasiello-Vailas, 1983).

Despite their problems, George and Nancy form a dyad and collaborate to support health-related self-care and avoid medical errors. George often assists Nancy in reading the prescriptions and being certain that she takes the right medications, as her failing eyesight makes this a difficult task. Similarly, Nancy helps George with his oxygen tanks and other strenuous tasks, given his limited mobility. Neither George nor Nancy could manage their health care alone, but together, they can manage as they continue to live independently. Finally, Pamela becomes an important outside resource for this health-care dyad when George and Nancy are faced with complex health communications and decisions.

SUMMARY

Older adults are prone to medical errors due to decreases in cognitive function, whereas middle-aged adults may make medical self-management errors due to their engaged, busy lifestyle. Providing older adults with information that can be processed at home decreases misunderstandings that lead to medical errors. Additionally, it is important not to present older adults with repeated statements about how something is not true because over time, it is likely that they will come to believe the false statement to be true due to its familiarity, rather than if they never heard it before. Adults at the oldest ages are most prone to medical errors due to cognitive decline. A variety of environmental supports are available and can be designed to reduce misunderstandings and medical self-care errors.

REFERENCES

Baddeley, A. (1994). Working memory: The interface between memory and cognition. In D. L. Schacter & E. Tulving (Eds.), *Memory systems* (pp. 351–368). Cambridge, MA: MIT Press.

Baltes, P. B., & Lindenberger, U. (1997). Emergence of a powerful connection between sensory and cognitive functions across the adult life span: A new window to the study of cognitive aging? *Psychology and Aging, 12,* 12–21.

Begg, I. M., Anas, A., & Farinacci, S. (1992). Dissociation of processes in belief: Source recollection, statement familiarity, and the illusion of truth. *Journal of Experimental Psychology: General, 121,* 446–458.

Bergman, U., & Wiholm, B. (1981). Patient medication on admission to medical clinic. *European Journal of Clinical Pharmacology, 20,* 85.

Botelho, R. J., & Dudrak, R. (1992). Home assessment of adherence to long-term medication in the elderly. *Journal of Family Practice, 35,* 61–65.

Brown, S., & Park, D. C. (in press). Memory for familiar and unfamiliar medical information in old and young adults. *Educational Gerontology.*

Craik, F. I. M., Anderson, N. D., Kerr, S. A., & Li, K. Z. H. (1995). Memory changes in normal ageing. In A. D. Baddeley, B. A. Wilson, & F. N. Watts (Eds.), *Handbook of memory disorders* (pp. 211–241). New York: Wiley.

Craik, F. I. M., Byrd, M., & Swanson, J. M. (1987). Patterns of memory loss in three elderly samples. *Psychology and Aging, 2,* 79–86.

Craik, F. I. M., & Jennings, J. M. (1992). Human memory. In F. I. M. Craik & T. A. Salthouse (Eds.), *The handbook of aging and cognition.* Hillsdale, NJ: Lawrence Erlbaum Associates.

Doherty, W. J., Schrott, H. B., Metcalf, L., & Iasiello-Vailas, L. (1983). The effects of spouse support and health beliefs on medication adherence. *Journal of Family Practice, 17,* 837–841.

Gilbert, D. T., Krull, D. S., & Malone, P. S. (1990). Unbelieving the unbelievable: Some problems in the rejection of false information. *Journal of Personality and Social Psychology, 59,* 601–613.

Green, L. W., Mullen, P. D., & Stainbrook, G. L. (1986). Programs to reduce drug errors in the elderly: Direct and indirect evidence from patient education. *Journal of Geriatric Drug Therapy, 1,* 59–70.

Hasher, L., Goldstein, D., & Toppino, T. (1977). Frequency and the conference of referential validity. *Journal of Verbal Learning and Verbal Behavior, 16,* 107–112.

Jacoby, L. L. (1999). Ironic effects of repetition: Measuring age-related differences in memory. *Journal of Experimental Psychology: Learning, Memory, and Cognition, 25,* 3–22.

Jacoby, L. L., & Dallas, M. (1981). On the relationship between autobiographical memory and perceptual learning. *Journal of Experimental Psychology: General, 3,* 306–340.

Johnson, M. K., DeLeonardis, D. M., Hashtroudi, S., & Ferguson, S. A. (1995). Aging and single versus multiple cues in source monitoring. *Psychology and Aging, 10,* 507–517.

Kiernan, P. J., & Isaacs, J. B. (1981). Use of drugs by the elderly. *Journal of Research in Sociological Medicine, 74,* 196.

Law, S., Hawkins, S. A., & Craik, F. I. M. (1998). Repetition-induced belief in the elderly: Rehabilitating age-related memory deficits. *Journal of Consumer Research, 25,* 91–107.

Light, L. L. (1991). Memory and aging: Four hypotheses in search of data. *Annual Review of Psychology, 42,* 333–376.

Mandler, G. (1980). Recognizing: The judgment of previous occurrence. *Psychological Review, 87,* 252–271.

Meyer, B. J. F., Russo, C., & Talbot, A. (1995). Discourse comprehension and problem solving: Decisions about the treatment of breast cancer by women across the life span. *Psychology and Aging, 10,* 84–103.

Morrell, R, W., Park, D. C., & Poon, L. W. (1989). Quality of instructions on prescription drug labels: Effects on memory and comprehension in young and old adults. *The Gerontologist, 29,* 345–353.

Morrell, R. W., Park, D. C., Kidder, D. P. & Martin, M. (1997). Adherence to anti-hypertensive medications across the life span. *The Gerontologist, 37,* 609–619.

Mutter, S. A., Lindsey, S. E., & Pliske, R. M. (1995). Aging and credibility judgment. *Aging and Cognition, 2,* 89–107.

Park, D. C. (1992). Applied cognitive aging research. In F. I. M. Craik & T. A. Salthouse (Eds.), *Handbook of cognition and aging* (pp. 449–493). Mahwah, NJ: Lawrence Erlbaum Associates.

Park, D. C. (1994). Aging, cognition, and work. *Human Performance, 7,* 181–205.

Park, D. C. (1999). Aging and the controlled and automatic processing of medical information and medical intentions. In Park, D. C., Morrell, R. W., & Shifren, K. (Eds.), *Processing of medical information in aging patients: Cognitive and human factors perspectives* (pp. 3–22). Mahwah, NJ: Lawrence Erlbaum Associates.

Park, D. C. (2000). Basic mechanisms accounting for age-related decline in cognitive function. In D. C. Park & N. Schwarz (Eds.), *Aging and cognition: A student primer* (pp. 3–21). Philadelphia: Psychology Press.

Park, D. C., Eaton, T. A., Larson, E. A., & Palmer, H. T. (1994). Implementation and impact of the Patient Self-Determination Act. *Southern Medical Journal, 87,* 971–977.

Park, D. C., & Hall-Gutchess, A. (2000). Cognitive aging and every day life. In D. C. Park & N. Schwarz (Eds.), *Aging and cognition: A student primer* (pp. 217–232). Philadelphia: Psychology Press.

Park, D. C., Hertzog, C., Leventhal, H., Morrell, R. W., Leventhal, E., Birchmore, D., Martin, M., & Bennett, J. (1999). Medication adherence in rheumatoid arthritis patients: Older is wiser. *Journal of American Geriatrics Society, 47,* 172–183.

Park, D. C., & Jones, T. R. (1996). Medication adherence and aging. In A. D. Fiske & W. A. Rogers (Eds.), *Handbook of human factors and the older adult* (pp. 257–288). San Diego, CA: Academic Press.

Park, D. C., & Kidder, D. (1996). Prospective memory and medication adherence. In M. Brandimonte, G. Einstein, & M. McDaniel (Eds.), *Prospective memory: Theory and applications* (pp. 369–390). Mahwah, NJ: Lawrence Erlbaum Associates.

Park, D. C., Lautenschlager, G., Hedden, T., Davidson, N. S., Smith, A. D., & Smith, P. (2002). Models of visuospatial and verbal working memory across the adult life span. *Psychology and Aging, 17*(2), 299–320.

Park, D. C., & Mayhorn, C. B. (1996). Remembering to take medications: The importance of nonmemory variables. In D. Hermann, M. Johnson, C. McEvoy, C. Hertzog, & P. Hertel (Eds.), *Research on practical aspects of memory* (Vol. 2, pp. 95–110). Mahwah, NJ: Lawrence Erlbaum Associates.

Park, D. C., Morrell, R. W., Frieske, D., Blackburn, A. B., & Birchmore, D. (1991). Cognitive factors and the use of over-the-counter medication organizers by arthritis patients. *Human Factors, 31*(3), 57–67.

Park, D. C., Morrell, R. W., Frieske, D., & Kincaid, D. (1992). Medication adherence behaviors in older adults: Effects of external cognitive supports. *Psychology and Aging, 7,* 252–256.

Park, D. C., Shifren, K., & Morrell, R. (1998, August). *Medication adherence in African Americans with hypertension.* San Francisco: American Psychological Association.

Park, D. C., Smith, A. D., Lautenschlager, G., Earles, J., Frieske, D., Zwahr, M., & Gaines, C. (1996). Mediators of long term memory performance across the lifespan. *Psychology and Aging, 11*(4), 621–637.

Richardson, M. A., Simons-Morton, B., & Annegers, J. F. (1993). Effect of perceived barriers on compliance with antihypertensive medication. *Health Education Quarterly, 20,* 489–503.

Salthouse, T. A. (1996). The processing-speed theory of adult age differences in cognition. *Psychological Review,103,* 403–428.

Schwartz, D., Wand, M., Zeitz, L., & Goss, M. E. (1962). Medication errors made by elderly chronically ill patients. *American Journal of Public Health, 52,* 2018–2029.

Skurnik, I., Park, D. C., & Schwarz, N. (2000, April). *Repeated warnings about false medical information can make it seem true: A paradoxical age difference.* Paper presented at the Eighth Cognitive Aging Conference, Atlanta, Georgia.

Spencer, W. D., & Raz, N. (1995). Differential effects of aging on memory for content and context: A meta-analysis. *Psychology and Aging, 10,* 527–539.

Zwahr, M. D., Park, D. C., & Shifren, K. (1999). Judgments about estrogen replacement therapy: The role of age, cognitive abilities and beliefs. *Psychology and Aging, 14,* 179–191.

Zwahr, M. D., Park, D. C., Eaton, T. A., & Larson, E. (1997). Implementation of the Patient Self-Determination Act: A comparison of nursing homes to hospitals. *Journal of Applied Gerontology, 16,* 190–207.

12 Prescription for Error: Can Health Care Providers Really "Do No Harm"?

Kenneth Dandurand
Clinical Pharmacy Associates, Inc.

> . . . for it remains true that those things which make us human
> are curiously, always close at hand.
>
> —Walt Kelly, "Pogo Looks at the Abominable
> Snowman." *The Funnies* (p. 292)

Walt Kelly was a satirist and political cartoonist most famous for his cartoon *Pogo,* published in newspapers across the country during the 1960s and 1970s. Although this particular quote is part of his assessment of pollution in the United States, it can be interpreted as addressing how we humans cope with other aspects of life, such as the context in which people work and our potential to make mistakes. The constantly changing circumstances surrounding health care create many and varied opportunities for error that people must routinely address. For this discussion, the people are health care professionals, physicians, pharmacists, and nurses; the context is the setting in which they provide care by prescribing, dispensing, and administering medications. This chapter presents four cases involving physicians, pharmacists, nurses, and patients in both hospital and ambulatory settings. These cases depict diverse circumstances in which drugs are prescribed and given, and issues that health care professionals encounter in striving to provide care that follows the Hippocratic guideline to do no harm.

GASTROINTESTINAL SPECIALIST, DR. YODER
PHARMACIST, MR. RANDAL

Marti Jones is a young woman with a 20-year history of irritable bowel syndrome (IBS), a disease that can be severely debilitating with frequent bouts of uncontrollable diarrhea and abdominal cramping. She also suffers from gastroesophageal reflux disease (GERD), in which acid from the stomach backs up into the throat and esophagus and creates a painful burning sensation. As a result of these health problems, Marti takes a number of medications including an antispasmodic to reduce gastrointestinal (GI) secretions, antimotility medication to reduce bowel movements, and an antihistaminic drug to block excess acid production. These drugs help her maintain generally stable bowel and stomach functioning. In addition to these drugs, Marti also takes prescription medication for other, unrelated health problems.

Normal hormone fluctuations, as well as the type and volume of food consumed, affect patients with IBS such as Marti. Because of this, management by drug therapy and control of food intake is essential to avoid the painful symptoms of this disease. Marti has become adept at this delicate balancing act by adjusting the dose and timing of medication while carefully controlling food intake. She routinely sees two physicians, an internist, Dr. Elder, for her general health needs and a GI specialist affiliated with a teaching hospital, Dr. Yoder, for her IBS and GERD conditions.

Marti was having more frequent GI discomfort than usual and was concerned about the impact of upcoming international travel on her bowel function. She consulted Dr. Elder, who sensed her anxiety and referred her to Dr. Yoder to fine-tune her medications to avoid problems during travel. Dr. Yoder elected to treat Marti's GERD symptoms aggressively, to help relieve her increased GI discomfort, for a short time prior to the trip by prescribing a four-fold increase in the acid-blocking medication she was taking. In addition, he added a potent anti-diarrhea agent to her regimen.

Marti took the new prescriptions to her local pharmacy to be filled. The pharmacist, Mr. Randal, was familiar with Marti's prescriptions and noted the changes in her medications, but decided not to phone Dr. Yoder to ask about the high dose of the new acid-blocking prescription. Having dispensed this dose to another patient recently, Mr. Randal was not inclined to question the use for Marti. Also, he was very busy with a sizable backlog of prescriptions to fill. Marti had received both drugs previously, so Mr. Randal presumed she knew of the side effects and did not specifically caution her about them.

Two days after starting the new prescriptions, Marti experienced disabling episodes of severe diarrhea and cramping. She promptly stopped the new drug ther-

apies prescribed by Dr. Yoder and started her previous drug therapy. Her bowel function returned to its usual state of balance. A friend referred Marti to a clinical pharmacist, Dr. Schultz, regarding the problems she experienced with Dr. Yoder's drug therapy. Dr. Schultz explained that the high dose of the acid blocker is five times more likely to cause diarrhea than her previous lower dose and resulted in the disruption of her delicate balance between medication and food intake.

Although the outcome from Marti's new drug therapies was not catastrophic, Marti is concerned that a similar response to a drug therapy could happen with more of an adverse outcome. She wants to avoid that painful experience in the future.

Issues

Marti Jones' experience highlights three issues frequently associated with medication adverse events: lack of drug knowledge, lack of patient information, and lack of communication (Leape et al., 1995). Among the most difficult challenges faced today by health care providers is not only keeping up with rapidly expanding medical information, but also integrating it into daily practice. Published clinical trials are, by design, tightly controlled and do not reflect variations in patients, disease, and other therapies that are the norm in everyday medical practice. Even if Dr. Yoder and Mr. Randal were aware that the acid blocker could cause diarrhea, they may not have been aware of the increased likelihood of GI disturbance with the use of large doses of this medication.

In a busy practice setting, it may be difficult to regularly find time to keep current with drug information and integrate it into the storehouse of knowledge used in clinical practice. Conversely, it is difficult when treating certain symptoms to recall all of the practical experience a professional has gained and link the new, published information to it. Dr. Yoder may have used this dose of acid blocker previously in 15 patients without the problems Marti experienced, but this small number of patients and particular patient characteristics can hide the true incidence of the GI problems that the drug can cause.

The amount of information in medicine is mind-boggling. In a typical month, over 34,000 published articles are added to the National Library of Medicine's database (Arndt, 1992); many of the articles are related to drug therapy. It is not surprising that practitioners find it difficult to keep current with the latest information. Fueled by the rapid increase in drug research and development by the pharmaceutical industry, more drugs are entering the market than ever before. The number of new drugs approved by the Food and Drug Administration more than doubled between 1992 and 1996. Since 1996, more than 30 new therapeutic chemical entities or reformulated products became available each year for use. Learning about three new drugs a month and integrating that information into existing knowledge is a formidable task for physicians and pharmacists.

Both Dr. Yoder's and Mr. Randal's situations exemplify the difficulty in practicing in a context that has deficits in patient information. They were not fully aware of all details of Marti's medical conditions. That is not necessarily their fault; patients often consult several physicians and have prescriptions filled by different pharmacies. Thus, primary care providers and specialist physicians as well as pharmacists are unaware of the panoply of medications and treatments a patient may be receiving. Despite the increased reliance on computers and information technology, in most cases there is no single place where all patient information resides nor is there viable integration of patient and drug knowledge databases (Dwyer, 1999).

Health care reimbursement and practice changes make the time-consuming effort of eliciting a full patient history during each episode of care virtually impossible. Compounding this is the difficulty of patients themselves recalling the details of all their medical issues. Therefore, critical patient information may be inaccessible at the point of care. Had additional information been available regarding Marti's health, Mr. Randal would have had a basis, in her past difficulties with controlling bowel movements, for questioning Dr. Yoder's dosing of the specific medication.

Communication difficulties among health professionals are frequently observed (Stanchfield, Lineoln, & Schafer, 1993), partly because caregivers operate in loosely defined and designed settings (Lawrence, 1999). Mr. Randal's pharmacy is located in Marti's town, whereas Dr. Yoder practices in the clinic at the teaching hospital 50 miles away. Even in local practice, pharmacists and physicians infrequently and ineffectively communicate regarding patients' drug therapy other than the 4×5-inch prescription paper. Although adding the patient diagnosis or indication for the drug therapy on the prescription is advocated (National Coordinating Council for Medication Error Reporting and Prevention [NCCMERP], 1996) as a method to improve communication between practitioners and reduce errors, this is infrequently done in the practice setting.

Sometimes questioning a particular medication order can be misconstrued as practicing outside the pharmacist's area of expertise rather than as an effort to clarify and improve treatment. As a result, Mr. Randal is hesitant to contact Dr. Yoder to question the high dose for fear of creating an adversarial situation. Although Dr. Yoder's office will send a report regarding his treatment to Marti's internist, it will take several weeks to reach Dr. Elder's office, let alone be reviewed. Rather than clarify the order with Dr. Yoder, Mr. Randal fills the prescription and gives it to Marti under the assumption that it must be reasonable because Dr. Yoder is the specialist.

PEDIATRIC NIGHT NURSE, PAULA PETERS
PHARMACIST, JOAN JOHNSON
RESIDENT PHYSICIAN, JANE HOWARD, M.D.

In a 100-bed community hospital, Paula Peters, a pediatric nurse on her third consecutive 12-hour night shift, calls and wakes Dr. Jane Howard, the resident physician in her first year of practice following medical school, who is on call, at 6 a.m. because Mark, a 2-year old immunosuppressed patient, spiked a temperature of 104°F. Mark has a multitude of health problems that require invasive medical interventions including intubation (placing a tube in his trachea, windpipe, that is attached to a ventilator) to help him breathe. Over the last 2 days, intravenous lines have been placed to supply him with life-sustaining fluid and electrolytes. Paula suspects that Mark has developed a nosocomial (hospital acquired) infection. Such an infection requires immediate action because it can be life threatening and difficult to treat.

Dr. Howard orders blood cultures for Mark to determine the type of infection. With that information, she can prescribe a course of treatment appropriate to the specific type of infection. She requests that the blood cultures be collected and processed along with previously ordered a.m. (morning) laboratory tests to determine the degree of Mark's renal function as well as the amount of his electrolytes and glucose. As soon as Paula hangs up from taking the order from Dr. Howard, the mother of another patient asks her to check her child's heat monitor that is beeping. Fifteen minutes later, Paula finds time to transcribe Dr. Howard's telephone order from where she had written it on a pad by the telephone to Mark's chart. At 6:30 a.m. Dr. Howard arrives on the floor, signs the telephone order for the blood tests on Mark's chart as required by hospital policy, and writes additional orders for antibiotics to be given. She does not specify on the order when the antibiotics are to be given; she presumes it to be understood that the condition of the patient is serious, and that antibiotics are to be given as soon as possible.

Paula's shift ends at 7:30 a.m. when Samantha Smothers, the day nurse, begins her shift. During morning report at shift change, Paula tells Samantha that she is waiting for the blood cultures to be taken with the a.m. labs that according to hospital policy are done at 8 a.m. Paula explains that because the hospital pharmacy does not open until 8 a.m., she has placed a copy of the antibiotic order to be filled for Mark in the bin at the nursing station for pick-up by the pharmacist, Joan Johnson, on her morning rounds. Unfortunately, Joan does not participate in this day's morning report because she is busy preparing two intravenous orders that are needed immediately for a patient in the intensive care unit and so is unaware that the labs had not been taken. Finally, Joan picks up the orders for Mark at 9 a.m. and, noticing by the time documented on the chart that the antibiotic orders were written at 6:30 a.m., she assumes that the nurses have made the antibiotics and administered them to the patient prior to the pharmacy opening.

Dr. Howard returns at 10 a.m. to check Mark and her other patients. She writes additional orders for a chest x-ray for Mark to rule out the possibility of pneumonia. Samantha discusses Mark's treatment with Dr. Howard; they note that the antibiotics have not been started. Dr. Howard then writes in Mark's chart "start antibiotics ordered at 6:30 a.m. STAT" (immediately) and "draw blood cultures if not already done." Samantha determines that the blood cultures were drawn at 8:40; she cannot understand the delay in receiving the antibiotics for Mark. She angrily calls Joan in the pharmacy to find out what happened to the antibiotics. The ensuing argument between Joan and Samantha over why the antibiotics were not given earlier is unproductive. Joan dispenses the antibiotics; Samantha administers a dose to Mark at 12 noon. Mark's condition deteriorates over the next 24 hours; fortunately, he recovers and is discharged after a 3-week hospital stay.

Issues

As in the previous case, there was a lack of effective communication between the health care providers. Despite working in the same physical environment of the hospital, opportunities abound that prevent optimal coordination of care between the physician, nurse, and pharmacist. The disparate duties of each professional are affected by a variety of circumstances and distractions that lead to a break in the continuity of care. Thus the logical anticipated process of taking the blood culture followed by giving the antibiotic shortly thereafter evolves into a series of assumptions and actions resulting in a serious delay in optimal care giving—a failure to connect the dots.

The chain of events starts with Dr. Howard's initial order for the blood culture given over the phone to Paula Peters, the night nurse. This lack of face-to-face contact precludes information transfer via multiple cues. Details could have been omitted, forgotten, or misunderstood during the telephone transfer of the order—details that were perpetuated on Mark's chart. Verbal orders should be used only when absolutely necessary (American Society of Health-System Pharmacists [ASHP], 1993; NCCMERP, 1996; American Academy of Pediatrics, 1998). As a safeguard against errors when verbal orders are necessary, the caregiver receiving the order should immediately write down the order and read it back for verification. Using computers for direct physician order entry is proposed to help eliminate this type of problem (Bates et al., 1998; Nold, 1997) but that is not in widespread use today.

In addition to communication, coordination between health care team members is crucial in avoiding errors. Due to historical, financial, and staffing considerations and the assumption that fewer duties are required on the night shift, many hospitals decide against staffing a night pharmacy. Although overall staff workload may be less during the night, patient needs dictate that the complement of professional staffing including the availability of pharmacists on the nightshift is critical (American Hospital Association [AHA], 1999). Coordination of professional services is contingent on access; that is, nurses cannot give the medication ordered by the physician unless they make it themselves if a pharmacist is not available to fill the order or review the order for potential problems. Not only is coordination affected but also there is a lack of checks and balances that the various health professionals provide to ensure that the medication orders are correct. Thus, organizational policies that increase workload and close the pharmacy during the night created significant gaps in effective communication that led to Mark not receiving the antibiotics as ordered.

Individuals working long shifts for extended days are prone to making mistakes (Kreuger, 1994). Because of the reduced staff on the night shift, Paula was providing care for more than the typical number of patients; her attention to any one patient was distracted by her duties for the others. When she phoned Dr. Howard, she was near the end of her shift, tired, and overextended by her excessive patient load and the long shift. She was not able to anticipate that Dr. Howard was not aware of the 8 a.m. labs policy. As shown in Fig. 12.1, the 6 a.m. order clearly specifies taking the blood levels with the morning labs; however, as

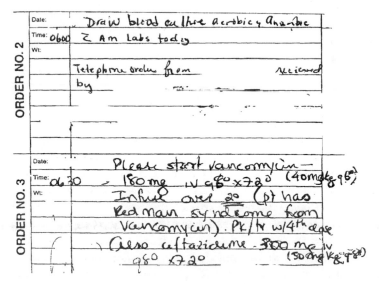

FIG. 12.1.   Confusing orders as depicted above allow for misinterpretation.

is the case in many health care organizations, there is a disconnect between policies and actual procedures.

Because of the multitude of health care providers with different professional and personal norms, situations like this are not always handled in the same manner. Thus Paula did not inform Dr. Howard that despite the concern for Mark's condition, the antibiotics would not be given to Mark until the cultures were taken, knowing that this would interfere with interpretation of this test. The 5 a.m. phone call that disrupted Dr. Howard's sleep, when she had only slept 45 minutes after being called to care for another patient, compromised her ability to realize that by requesting the cultures for morning labs, there would be a delay in administering Mark's antibiotics.

When Joan Johnson, the pharmacist, began her day, she was immediately distracted by urgent orders to fill medications for another patient, preventing her from participating in that morning's patient care rounds. The lack of a night pharmacist prevented an appropriate exchange of information and led her to assume the antibiotics were made and given to Mark by the nurse.

ATTENDING PHYSICIAN, DR. WANG
CONSULTING NEUROLOGIST, DR. SINGH

Mr. Jones is an 80-year-old patient with a variety of ailments including congestive heart failure (CHF), stomach ulcers, kidney disease, arthritis, and hypertension. At home he takes eight prescription drugs including a beta-blocking agent that helps lower his blood pressure and three over-the-counter and two herbal alternative medications. His CHF worsened; he was admitted to the hospital and placed on diuretics to reduce fluid build-up in his body and the medication digoxin to strengthen the heart pumping. He also was given a beta-blocking drug that was different from the one he was taking at home. During his hospitalization Mr. Jones had seizures. The attending physician, Dr. Wang, intended to write an order for 100 mg twice daily of Cerebryx, a new drug for seizure control; however, he inadvertently wrote the order for 100 mg twice daily of Celebrex, a drug to treat arthritis.

The pharmacist dispensed Celebrex as ordered and the nurse administered it for 2 days, assuming that Dr. Wang was treating Mr. Jones' arthritis. Mr. Jones continued to have mild seizures. Because of the seizures, Dr. Singh, a consulting neurologist, reviewed Mr. Jones' chart and discovered that Celebrex had been ordered and given to Mr. Jones instead of Cerebryx. After 2 weeks on Cerebryx, the seizures subsided and Mr. Jones' cardiac function gradually improved. He was discharged on the medications started in the hospital, including the new beta-blocker with a handful of papers with instructions on his medications.

Mr. Jones returned home and took the new medications as directed, as well as resuming the medications he had been taking prior to his hospitalization, including the original beta-blocker. One week after returning home, Mr. Jones died of heart failure as a result of the additive effect of the two beta-blockers combined with his medical condition.

Issues

Although poor handwriting (Winslow, Nestor, Davidoff, Thompson, & Borum, 1997) and transcription practices represent major factors in medication errors, factors outside the immediate caregiver–patient setting also can play a large role in mishaps. Brand names that manufacturers assign to various drugs prior to their marketing can be very similar both in appearance and pronunciation to brand names of other drugs. Because of this, Dr. Wang's writing an order for Celebrex when intending to write Cerebryx was an error waiting to happen. Although clearly written (Fig. 12.2), the similar-sounding name and dosage made it difficult for the nurse or pharmacist to pick up this discrepancy.

Remarkably, there is no coordination on assigning names to new drugs, which often are similar (Cohen, 1995). Brand naming by manufacturers is done primarily to enhance name recognition and marketing. The drugs Celebrex and Cerebryx are used for different indications; however, the similarity of names easily can lead to substitution. Such substitution may not be readily noted because the patient may have the indications for the substituted drug. This happened with Mr. Jones, who had arthritis, so the nurses and pharmacist assumed that the Celebrex was ordered to treat this condition. Also, because another drug

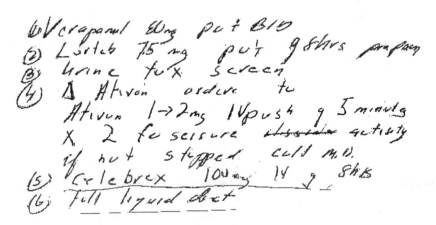

FIG. 12.2.   Example of clearly written order for the wrong drug with a similar sounding name and identical dosage.

(Ativan) was prescribed for immediate treatment of the seizures, the pharmacist and nurse did not suspect that Cerebryx was the intended drug.

It is evident that communication and coordination are critical links in medication-related error, especially when patients go from one health care setting to another. Mr. Jones was discharged with his new medications including the beta-blocker, but he received no clear explanation nor did he read the written material given him outlining the reasons for taking his new medications, which is not uncommon. Thus he was not aware that the new beta-blocker was not supposed to be taken with the beta-blocker he had at home. In addition, he received no explicit instructions to discontinue taking his previous medicines; he did what he thought was right. Back in the comfort of his own home, he resumed his routine and started back on his beta-blocker clearly unaware that this should be discontinued.

Mr. Jones was elderly. The elderly are particularly prone to ineffective communication with health professionals because of cognitive decline, hearing losses, and external factors such as gender role that would preclude a man asking questions (Vroman, Cohen, & Volkman, 1994). In addition, medication use including self-medication with alternative medicinals increases as a person ages. Mr. Jones required multiple prescription drugs and used a variety of over-the-counter products. Such a combination can result in interactions and side effects that can cause confusion and difficulty managing a complicated regimen of when and why these agents are taken.

PHARMACIST, RON WHITE

Ron White works as a pharmacist for a large chain drug store in a mid-size city. He has been practicing for 3 years and works rotating day and evening shifts. The store where he works is staffed by one pharmacist and one assistant on each of two shifts (8 a.m. to 4 p.m. and 2 p.m. to 10 p.m.) with an overlap of the teams for 2 hours in the middle of the day. Between 300 and 400 prescriptions a day are filled during those two shifts. An additional pharmacist is available to help on Mondays and Thursdays, which typically are the busier days.

On a particularly busy Thursday at 11:30 a.m., Ron is having difficulty getting the computerized online payment system to accept a prescription for a child's antibiotic. The system rejects the payment, so Ron has no option but to present the mother with a bill for $109 for a 10-day course of the antibiotic. The mother is angry and argues that the child is covered under her plan. Ron places a call to the insurance company. After 10 minutes of talking with three people at the insurance company, Ron determines that the child is covered under the father's health plan and re-enters the prescription for approval. During this time, four patients have dropped off 15 new prescriptions to add to the 30

*called-in refills to be picked up later in the day. Ron is aware of the mounting
expectations of the patients to have their prescriptions filled quickly; this makes
him anxious and distracted as the work piles up.*

*For some patients, getting their prescriptions is the end of a long day of trav-
eling to the doctor's offices, many with sick children, waiting for their appoint-
ments, and traveling to the pharmacy. They tend to be impatient with delays,
wondering how long it could take to count out some pills. It is 12:30 p.m.; Ron
has been too busy for lunch and continues filling prescriptions, including one for
a blood-thinning drug with directions to take "5 mg as directed" from Dr. Smith
for Mrs. Bledsoe, a new patient.*

*Ron's partner, Brenda Smith, comes in at 2 p.m. and together they are able to
clean up the backlog of prescriptions, make several calls to physicians' offices
to obtain refills for patients who have requested them, and place an order to
replenish stock. Ron leaves at 5 p.m. having not eaten lunch and wondering if he
filled Mrs. Bledsoe's prescription with the proper dose of blood-thinning agent.
Later that day the nurse from Dr. Smith's office calls Mrs. Bledsoe and, based
on the results of laboratory tests, instructs her to take five of the blood-thinning
agent. Mrs. Bledsoe takes 5 tablets and is admitted to the hospital the next day
with disorientation.*

Issues

There is scant acknowledgment of the possible contribution of workload and
interruptions to error in pharmacies. Practitioners like Ron White can give only
a fixed amount of time and attention to the various tasks at hand; interruptions
can affect decision making and performance (Cook & Woods, 1994). When the
mother presented the prescription that was not accepted by the insurance company, Ron spent considerable time addressing the problem while additional prescriptions were constantly being brought in or called in to be filled. The result
was an ongoing effort to catch up by increasing the number of prescriptions
filled in the reduced available time. This is only one of many disruptions that
occurred during Ron's workday.

On a typical day Ron receives 30 phone calls from physicians' offices to take
verbal orders or clarify existing prescriptions, is asked repeatedly by customers
for help with over-the-counter products, and is asked to provide assistance and
advice to patients and technicians. Continuous interruptions while filling prescriptions disrupt his focus on the task at hand and increase the chance for error.
The lack of a routine explains why Ron, after he leaves his job, is uneasy about
the strength of blood-thinning agent he placed in Mrs. Bledsoe's prescription
bottle. Workload and disruptions also are prominent factors that impact the performance of nurses and physicians in the health care setting.

The prescription for Mrs. Bledsoe presents two additional factors that can foster medication error. The "as directed" instructions are vague and rely on the patient recalling the physician's instructions or are dependent on other patient-related factors that must be present, such as waiting for the physician's office to call with directions based on lab results or patient interpretation of symptoms. "As directed" also does not allow for a check by the pharmacist because he is unaware of the intended use, thus removing a safety net in the medication use process (Anonymous, 1996).

As illustrated by this case, Mrs. Bledsoe is directed to take a certain amount of this prescription for blood thinning based on laboratory results relayed to her by Dr. Smith's office later that day. Even though this process was explained when she was given the prescription, it is likely that "taking five" means 5 mg or one tablet to the nurse relaying the instructions; however, Mrs. Bledsoe interprets the instructions to take five tablets. The resulting overdose occurs without Ron's knowledge so he is unable to clarify and prevent the mishap.

SYSTEMS FACTORS

The typical response to an adverse outcome in health care is to blame the care provider most closely associated with the patient and the outcome in time and space. The real-world stories depicted in this chapter illustrate factors from the perspectives of the health care providers that contribute directly or indirectly to inappropriate medication therapy. This indicates that blaming the care provider is attacking the symptom rather than the problem.

Marti Jones received medication that exacerbated her problem. Mr. Randal, the pharmacist, is a ready candidate for being blamed for the error of filling and giving Marti a prescription that was four times the usual dose with the potential to exacerbate her medical condition. Blame and possible remedial action against Mr. Randal or Dr. Yoder would not prevent a similar occurrence because the dose may be appropriate for some patients. If an accurate history is not available, health care professionals have no option but to use the patient and drug information available to them at the point of service; errors can simply indicate unavailable information.

Although modern medicine has become more diligent in approving drugs and removing those that show little or no efficacy, the increased reliance on drug therapy as the primary treatment course of most illnesses exposes patients to significant potential harm as well as benefit. It has long been established that the United States is the world leader in the number of prescriptions per capita (Venulet, 1975). This particularly is true at the beginning of the 21st century. The rapid rate of new drug development and related clinical information has greatly outstripped the ability of health care providers to keep pace with the knowledge requirements to optimally use drug therapy and avoid mistakes.

Communication and Coordination

The most common error-provoking conditions that occur in the use of medications revolve around the inability to access information (Leape et al., 1995). This is a result, partly, of inaccurate and insufficient databases of both drug and patient information sources (Jollis et al., 1993; Nold, 1997). In addition, practitioners have difficulty using electronic databases because of lack of experience, training, or time (Davidoff & Florance, 2000). Other reasons for the inability to access information are the lack of the effective communication and coordination required by health care professionals directing patient care through a maze of practice settings and treatment options. Examples of this appear in all the stories presented in this chapter. Paula Peters, the night nurse, and Joan Johnson, the pharmacist, each expected the other to prepare the antibiotic for the patient. Dr. Wang inadvertently wrote orders for a drug that has a very similar name to the intended drug. Miscommunication occurred between the nurse and Mrs. Bledsoe regarding the number of tablets to be taken. The constant thread in all these situations is there is no clear, unequivocal mechanism that promotes timely and accurate communication and coordination.

Practitioners rely on the conventions at hand, such as "take as directed." At first glance, it appears easier to write a prescription for Mrs. Bledsoe with the instructions "take as directed" and periodically follow her laboratory blood tests and adjust the dose over the phone. Those instructions could cause difficulty, however, when Mrs. Bledsoe takes an incorrect dose of the medication from the beginning of the dose cycle and the laboratory tests are performed at a much later date. In this instance, the convention "take as directed" is an incident waiting to happen.

For cultural, educational, or cognitive reasons, communication often becomes difficult (Vroman, Cohen, & Volkman, 1994). It is understandable, then, that Mr. Jones is unclear whether he should continue his home medication when he is discharged from the hospital. Despite what physicians believe, the majority of patients are unclear about instructions at discharge from the hospital (Calkins et al., 1997). Reprimanding the caregivers in these cases would do little to prevent future mishaps.

An interdisciplinary health care team approach improves communication and coordination and more significantly, patient care (Baggs et al., 1999; Leape et al., 1999; Monson, Bond, & Schuna, 1981; Montazeri & Cook, 1994; Zimmerman et al., 1993). Despite the known benefits of team-directed care with regular and receptive collaboration, the reality in health care is that this concept is not the normative practice (Lawrence, 1999; Ray, 1998). An obvious example of noncommunication because of a lack of teamwork occurred with Paula Peters, Dr. Howard, Joan Johnson, and Samantha Smothers regarding Mark's anti-biotic—a lack that was due to a number of factors such as workload.

Workload

Many industries such as nuclear power and chemical processing place limits on the amount of work an individual can do in a specified period of time. This seems reasonable in terms of risk to the operator and to the quality of the product or service delivered. Contrary to this, workload limits are rarely set on the delivery of medical care. Ron White, the pharmacist, and his partner, Brenda Smith, fill an average of 400 prescriptions a day. Although they have assistants to help with their dispensing activities, spending as little as 5 minutes per prescription would require 33 man-hours per day to fill 400 prescriptions. This time includes checking, filling, billing, clarifying orders with physicians, reviewing new orders, and consulting with patients. The ambulatory prescription drug market alone has grown approximately 50% since 1992, approaching 3 billion prescriptions dispensed in 1998 (Somnath, 1998). In contrast to the number of prescriptions, the number of pharmacists has increased by only 12% from 1996 through 1999. This suggests that workload will continue to increase.

In hospitals, the change from fee-for-service to a fixed payment model as exemplified by Medicare payments can increase the amount and the intensity of workload for health care professionals (Applegate, 1994). Paula Peters, on the night shift, may have to care for up to 10 patients and must regularly triage (care for patients in the order of the seriousness of their problem—the most serious patient first) to prioritize her work. Although excessive workload typically is not considered as inducing error in health care, health care workers themselves rank workload as a factor that contributes to error (Serig, 1994).

Policies and Rules

Failure to follow organizational rules and policies frequently is a cause of medication errors (Leape et al., 1995). Add to this the overlap and inconsistencies in policies developed by individual departments in health care (Laine, Galt, Langford, Prout, & Puckett, 1994) and it is not surprising to find that rules are frequently broken. Dr. Howard's intention of starting the antibiotics for Mark as soon as possible conflicted with her order for taking the blood culture with morning labs because of the policy of defining morning labs to be done at 8 a.m. Both Paula Peters and Dr. Howard clinically were aware that the patient's blood cultures needed to be taken before the antibiotics are given. Nonetheless, Paula followed the order written by Dr. Howard, who was not aware of the dilemma the 8 a.m. policy caused. The inability to consistently interpret and apply workable procedures causes increased variability in delivering care, resulting in an increased potential for error.

Social and Organizational Decision Making

Pressures from outside the immediate work setting are often placed on health care professionals and can lead to mishaps. These include legal, economic, political, and management decision making. Managers may decide staffing patterns based on economics rather than need. Thus the unavailability of a night pharmacist and only one nurse caring for a large number of patients are decisions made outside the actual patient-care arena that compromised the ability of Paula Peters, the night nurse, to avoid errors. She did not have tools and resources necessary for a fail-safe work environment. The arguing of Samantha Smothers, the day nurse, and Joan Johnson, the pharmacist, points to a lack of leadership in creating a continuous improvement approach to handling such errors (Batalden & Stoltz, 1993). Indicative of this is a lack of integration of responsibilities and values with the work being conducted. The organization replaces trust with an atmosphere of fear (Ryan, 1999) and further confounds the efforts of practitioners to improve the conditions in which they work.

CONCLUSIONS

There are many lessons to learn from the four cases and the circumstances surrounding them that contributed to error. The actions of a health care provider can directly cause an error; however, the source of such actions is the reasonable target for remediation. There are a multitude of circumstances and system issues including the complexity of prescribing, dispensing, administering, and monitoring medication that contribute to medication errors. To reduce errors, those circumstances and issues must be identified and addressed.

The stories presented in this chapter represent only a small portion of the situations in which health care providers and patients interact. Nonetheless, those stories provide a glimpse of the difficulties that face practitioners like Dr. Yoder, Nurse Paula Peters, and Pharmacist Ron White on a day-to-day basis in a variety of settings. The inability to prevent harm to patients like Mark, Mr. Jones, and Mrs. Bledsoe, reflected in these stories, has less to do with the capabilities of the practitioners and more to do with the systems factors that they constantly encounter. Although the majority of health care interactions involving medication are safe and effective, error-provoking systems factors lead to incidents. It is beyond human ability, particularly the ability of a stressed and fatigued health care provider, to anticipate and compensate for all such factors; to reduce error, the factors must be changed.

REFERENCES

American Academy of Pediatrics. (1998). Prevention of medication errors in the pediatric inpatient setting (RE9751). *Pediatrics, 102,* 428–430.

American Hospital Association. (1999). Successful practices for improving medication safety, Retrieved from www.aha.org/medicationsafety/medicalsafety20015.asp.

American Society of Health-System Pharmacists. (1993). Guidelines on preventing medication errors in hospitals. *American Journal of Hospital Pharmacists, 50,* 305–314.

Anonymous. (1996). Top priority actions for preventing adverse drug events in hospitals. Recommendations of an expert panel. *American Journal of Health-System Pharmacists, 53,* 747–751.

Applegate, M. H. (1994). Diagnosis related groups: Are patients in jeopardy. In M. S. Bogner (Ed.), *Human error in medicine* (pp. 349–371). Hillsdale, NJ: Lawrence Erlbaum Associates.

Arndt, K. A. (1992). Information excess in medicine overview relevance to dermatology, and strategies for coping. *Archives of Dermatology, 128*(9), 1249–1256.

Baggs, J. G., Schmitt, M. H., Mushlin, A. I., Mitchell, P. H., Eldredge, D. H., Oakes, D., & Hutson, A. D. (1999). Association between nurse–physician collaboration and patient outcomes in three intensive care units. *Critical Care Medicine, 27,* 1991–1998.

Batalden, P. B., & Stoltz, P. K. (1993). A framework for the continual improvement of health care: Building and applying professional and improvement knowledge to test changes in daily work. *Joint Commission Journal of Quality Improvement, 19,* 424–452.

Bates, D. W., Leape, L. L., Cullen, D. J., Laird, N., Petersen, L. A., Teich, J. M., Burdick, E., Hickey, M., Kleefield, S., Shea, B., Vander Vliet, M., & Seger, D. L. (1998). Effect of computerized physician order entry and a team intervention on prevention of serious medication errors. *Journal of the American Medical Association, 280,* 1311–1316.

Calkins, D. R., Davis, R. B., Reiley, P., Phillips, R. S., Pineo, K. L., Delbanio, T. L., & Lezoni, L. I. (1997). Patient–physician communication at hospital discharge and patient understanding of the postdischarge treatment plan. *Archives of Internal Medicine, 157,* 1026–1030.

Cohen, M. R. (1995). Drug product characteristics that foster drug-use-system errors. *American Journal of Health-System Pharmacists, 52,* 395–399.

Cook, R. I., & Woods, D. D. (1994). Operating at the sharp end: The complexity of human error. In M. S. Bogner (Ed.), *Human error in medicine* (pp. 255–310). Hillsdale, NJ: Lawrence Erlbaum Associates.

Davidoff, F., & Florance, V. (2000). The informationist: A new health profession? *Annals of Internal Medicine, 132,* 996–998.

Dwyer, C. (1999). Ideas and trends: Medical informatics and health care computing. *Annals of Internal Medicine, 130,* 170–172.

Jollis, J. G., Ancukiewicz, M., DeLong, E. R., Pryor, D. B., Muhlbaier, L. H., & Mark, D. B. (1993). Discordance of databases designed for claims payment versus clinical information systems. *Annals of Internal Medicine, 119,* 844–50.

Krueger, G. P. (1994). Fatigue, performance, and medical error. In M. S. Bogner (Ed.), *Human error in medicine* (pp. 311–326). Hillsdale, NJ: Lawrence Erlbaum Associates.

Laine, G. A, Galt, M. A., Langford, J. A., Prout, D. L., & Puckett, W. H., (1994). Hospitalwide medication policies and standards. *American Journal of Hospital Pharmacists, 51*, 2949–2951.

Lawrence, D. (1999). Is medical care obsolete? *Hospital Pharmacy, 12*, 1395–1400.

Leape, L. L., Bates, D. W., Cullen, D. J., Cooper, J., Demonaco, H. J. Gallivan, T., Hallisey, R., Ives, J., Laird, N., Laffel, G., Nemeskal, R., Petersen, L. A.., Porter, K., Servi, D., Shea, B. F., Small, S. D., Sweitzer, B. J., Thompson, B. T., & Vander Vliet, M. (1995). Systems analysis of adverse drug events. *Journal of the American Medical Association, 274*, 35–43.

Leape, L. L., Cullen, D. J., Clapp, M. D., Burdick, E., Demonaco, H. J., Erickson, J. I., & Bates, D. W. (1999). Pharmacist participation on physician rounds and adverse drug events in the intensive care unit. *Journal of the American Medical Association, 282*, 267–270.

Monson, R., Bond, C. A., & Schuna, A. (1981). Role of the clinical pharmacist in improving drug therapy. Clinical pharmacist in outpatient therapy. *Archives of Internal Medicine, 141*, 1441–1444.

Montazeri, M., & Cook, D. J. (1994). Impact of a clinical pharmacist in a multidisciplinary intensive care unit. *Critical Care Medicine, 22*, 1044–1048.

National Coordinating Council for Medication Error Reporting and Prevention: Council Recommendations. (1996, September 4). *Recommendations to correct error-prone aspects of prescription writing.* Press Release, NCCMERP.

Nold, E. G. (1997). Trends in health information technology. *American Journal of Health-System Pharmacists, 54*, 269–274.

Ray, M. D. (1998). Shared borders: Achieving the goals of interdisciplinary patient care. *American Journal of Health-System Pharmacists, 55*, 1369–1374.

Ryan, K. D. (1999). Driving fear out of the medication-use process so that improvement can occur. *American Journal of Health-System Pharmacists, 56*, 1765–1769.

Serig, D. I. (1994). Radiopharmaceutical misadministrations: What's wrong? In M. S. Bogner (Ed.), *Human error in medicine* (pp. 179–195). Hillsdale, NJ: Lawrence Erlbaum Associates.

Somnath, P. (1998). Trendwatch, Rx market shows healthy growth. *U.S. Pharmacist, 23*, 10.

Stanchfield, J., Lineoln, E., & Schafer, B. (1993). PIAA medication error study. *Physician Insurers Association of America*, 1–44.

Venulet, J. (1975). Increasing threat to man as a result of frequently uncontrolled and widespread use of various drugs. *International Journal of Clinical Pharmacology, 12*, 387–394.

Vroman, G., Cohen, I., & Volkman, N. (1994). Misinterpreting cognitive decline in the elderly: Blaming the patient. In M. S. Bogner (Ed.), *Human error in medicine* (pp. 93–122). Hillsdale, NJ: Lawrence Erlbaum Associates.

Winslow, E. H., Nestor, V. A., Davidoff, S. K., Thompson, P. G., & Borum, J. C. (1997). Legibility and completeness of physicians' handwritten medication orders. *Heart Lung, 26*, 158–164.

Zimmerman, J. E., Shortell, S. M., Rousseau, D. M., Duffy, J., Gillies, R. R., Knaus, W. A., Devers, K., Wagner, D. P., & Draper, E. A. (1993). Improving intensive care: Observations based on organizational studies in nine intensive care units: A prospective, multicenter study. *Critical Care Medicine, 10*, 1443–1451.

13 All the Men and Women Merely Players

Marilyn Sue Bogner
Institute for the Study of Human Error, LLC

All the world's a stage . . .

—William Shakespeare (1564–1616)
As You Like It, II: 7

The inside stories of the preceding 11 chapters present the perspectives from a variety of care providers of factors contributing to misadventures in health care. Most of those misadventures resulted in patients needing additional care, being injured, or dying. Some stories include descriptions of several events that barely missed causing an adverse outcome; some stories are of adverse events waiting to happen. Regardless of the outcome of the misadventure, the stories are rich in factors that impinge on and affect the behavior of the individual engaged in health care. As rich as the information in the inside stories is, the sheer quantity of it could present a data management problem.

Reports of adverse events typically have only a small fraction of the amount of information of the inside stories, and the focus typically is on the action of the provider that caused the adverse outcome, such as the act of administering the wrong medication to a patient. The recommendation regarding error reporting in the Institute of Medicine (IOM) report on error (Kohn, Corrigan, & Donaldson, 1999) is that standardized information should be collected. Descriptions of the causes of error from such error reporting activities can present a picture of error relatively divorced from the reality as represented by the detail in our stories. A lesson is to be learned about inferences from information from the fable of the blindfolded man and the elephant.

THE ELEPHANT OF ERROR

In the fable, a man who has never seen an elephant is blindfolded and asked to describe the elephant based on information he obtains from feeling the elephant with his hand. The man's hand is placed on the elephant's leg; from that information, he declares that the elephant is like a tree. The blindfolded man's hand then is placed on the elephant's trunk; from that information, he states he was wrong before, that the elephant resembles a serpent. When the blindfold is removed and the man sees the elephant, he is astounded and argues that such a creature could not be what he had felt. As information from touching the leg and the trunk of the elephant misleads the blindfolded man in describing the elephant, so information from of the various error-reporting activities might be misleading in describing the elephant of error. Reported errors categorized by problem and objective assessment provide examples.

Categorization by Problem

One way to identify factors that contribute to error is to determine the problem the care provider had that apparently caused an error—information typical of that collected by some error reporting activities. That information can be reviewed across errors to determine common problems. Review of the inside stories found three factors common to two or more error situations: information, equipment, and reimbursement.

Information.   Information as a factor in error is evident in: the absence of personal identification for an accident victim and the assignment of an identifier similar to that of another patient. This contributed to a blood bank technician releasing and a nurse transfusing the blood for the wrong patient (chapter 2). No information about the seriousness of the condition of an unidentified patient was provided to the Shock Trauma Center prior to the arrival of that patient. This hindered the assignment of appropriate personal to various tasks for that patient culminating in a medical student being assigned a task beyond his level of expertise (chapter 3). The conditions of two of the patients visited by the home health nurse deteriorated because in one case, a woman didn't know how to care for her spouse. In the other case, the patient didn't know how to use the equipment necessary to care for her health problem (chapter 10). An elderly woman did not assimilate information from her physician even though she appeared to the physician to do so (chapter 11). The pharmacist's lack of information about a patient's current medication led to filling a prescription that caused over-medication and subsequent gastric upset (chapter 12).

Equipment.   Equipment was a problem for a surgeon who had difficulties using the instruments in laparoscopic surgery and for a nurse who had to be careful not to fall over the clutter those instruments caused in the operating room (chapter 5). Another surgeon had similar difficulties with the instruments, which were even more of a problem because he was short and the operating table could not be lowered adequately. To perform the procedure, he had to stand and operate foot peddles for his instruments on a stepstool (chapter 6).

A vital signs monitor with an obscure indication that the alarm was disabled denied an anesthesiologist an important warning about the patient's condition (chapter 7). The erratic false alarms of the portable monitors were annoying, hence distracting to an anesthesiologist; in addition, that left-handed anesthesiologist had to contort herself to accommodate to a workstation designed for right-handed people (chapter 8). The pervasiveness of technology in the intensive care unit hindered the nurses' application of their clinical skills, which could lead to missing significant signals of deterioration in the condition of the patient (chapter 9).

Reimbursement.   Issues regarding reimbursement by health maintenance organizations (HMO) discouraged a surgeon from ordering a pre-surgery scan that could have provided important information for the surgical procedure (chapter 4). The home health nurse experienced significant stress because of time pressure resulting from spending considerable time finding a way to obtain needed supplies for a patient because that patient's HMO would not authorize payment as well as an inordinate amount of time arranging transportation to a nearby emergency room because the patient's HMO would authorize payment only for a distant facility in their network (chapter 10).

The Elephant of Categories of Error

The previously described consolidation of identified problems of error across cases and the identification of possible causes of error by a single term leads to macro-level responses. Examples of such responses are general efforts to train the providers to check for adequate information, enhance the provider's familiarity with equipment, and educate the providers on the fine points of HMO reimbursement policies.

It is acknowledged that it is expeditious to aggregate reported problems by category of error; however, such clustering eclipses the variety of forms of errors in a given category as is evident in the details in the situations that were the basis for assigning the categories. The responses by targeting a general problem would not address the eclipsed contextual factors that define the problem. Hence, rather than describing an elephant of error, inference from those consolidations of information describe an aardvark.

Objective Assessment

Objective assessment of error is conducted either directly or indirectly by an uninvolved person typically trained to assess according to some criteria. Such assessment can take many forms. One form is shadowing a care provider to observe his or her behavior. This has proven successful in analyzing and evaluating laparoscopic surgical processes for the purpose of designing new methods and instruments (Sjoerdsma, 1998), but it is too resource intensive to be practical for identifying errors.

Other forms of objective assessment, such as interviews and questionnaires, are developed by those who seek the information, such as researchers. The interview schedule and questions, although developed with the best of intentions for collecting valid and reliable information, are developed to meet the needs of the researcher. Information solicited by the questions may be unrelated to what actually provokes error. Even though the questions have been designed to represent the perspective of the care provider, the questions come from the perspective of the individual developing them; the information sought is filtered by that person's experience (Kelly, 1963) as well as subject to the researcher's subjective, pragmatic stop rules (Rasmussen, 1990) discussed in chapter 1.

Can these objective assessments tap into the factors that contributed to, induced, and provoked errors? Objective assessment often means an opinion by an expert; however, in the study of behavior, and error is behavior as discussed in chapter 1, to substitute such an opinion, regardless of the area of expertise, for the facts from the perspective of the individual involved in the error, is not objective, it is wrong (Lewin, 1942/1964b). Then how might the web of factors that contribute to error be untangled?

Describing the Elephant of Error by Analyzing an Adverse Event

The error-inducing properties of contextual factors are obvious in the descriptions of misadventures in heath care presented by the inside stories; however, determining such factors from analyzing a health care misadventure can be challenging. In working to meet that challenge it is important to keep in mind that the ultimate goal of analysis is not to assign responsibility solely to one factor because, as illustrated in the stories, many factors contribute to error and limited information can result in inaccurate conclusions as in the fable of the elephant.

Rather, the goal of error analysis is to determine why the error occurred in terms of factors that can be addressed and changed by those responsible for the factors to avoid recurrence of the error. When confronted with the task of untangling the web of error—more specifically, to identify, target, and effectively change factors that have contributed to an adverse event described solely as an information-related error—the analysis of the event should be performed in a manner to conserve and appreciate the nuances in the complexity of possible contributing factors such as those in the inside stories.

In analyzing an adverse event surrounding an error, it is difficult for a person addressing the error, who is not the person involved in the error, to know where to start because humans engage in many and varied behaviors when interacting with their environment and with other people. One of the major problems in identifying factors that contribute to adverse outcomes in health care is the myriad of factors, indeed an intricate, tangled web of factors that form the context of a misadventure.

UNTANGLING THE WEB OF ERROR

A two-pronged approach provides guidance in untangling the web and determining discrete error-provoking factors that can be targeted for remedial activities. One prong is an approach that introduces the important factor of time in describing the path to error. The other prong is a technique for increasing the scale of the map describing the path to error to life-size so the details of that path are more apparent. That technique, alluded to in chapter 1, is used by astute observers of the human condition, the technique employed in drama.

Typically error is considered as occurring at one point in time; indeed, that is how the act that precipitated the adverse outcome occurred; however, the influences that culminated in that act occurred otherwise. It is commonly acknowledged that an adverse outcome, an error, is not the result of the solitary precipitating act, but a cascade of errors (Gaba, 1994). Nonetheless, it is not common for the influence of an event that happened earlier to be included actively in addressing an error. An error can be the last domino knocked over when a column of dominos falls; considering it only as a fallen domino gives no information about the conditions that led to its fall. The purpose of the discussion of each of the two prongs is to demonstrate the importance of considering the column of dominos by expanding the reader's consideration of error.

Path to Error

As the journey toward a destination can take a variety of routes over a geographical terrain, there are a variety of possible paths leading to error. The terrain for those paths has a geological strata formed by the systems of the context of care described in chapter 1: the strata of ambient conditions, physical environment, social environment, organizational factors, and the bedrock of the legal-regulatory-reimbursement-national culture factors. That terrain is not smooth; at times there are rough spots such as a pothole exposing organizational factors, a ditch with a social environment bottom. The path along the terrain is defined by waypoints, error-related landmarks such as an incident caused by the pothole or a severe turn necessitated by a hill.

The care provider is the driver for the journey; the passengers are the means of providing care and care recipient. The critical element for the journey is the vehicle, the power source for the journey. The vehicle is an expanded version of the source of the inside stories, the perspective of the care provider. The basis for the expansion is a concept from psychology, that a person's behavior is driven not by all the factors surrounding him or her, but by those factors that influence the person at the time, factors in the person's life-space (Lewin, 1940/1964a).

The life-space of the individual consists of all facts that have existence and excludes those that do not have existence for the individual at a given time. A person's life-space is the driving force in his or her life; it influences that person's perspective as well as behavior. The concept of life-space is important because it addresses a factor that typically is omitted in considering error, the factor of time.

The life-space of a person is dynamic; it changes over time as it influences the person's behavior and is influenced by the reactions to that behavior by entities in the environment. The factors in a person's life-space that influence a person's behavior at a given point in time (Gold, 1999) are not restricted to those from that immediate context. The influence of life-space can represent factors from the past as well as those anticipated in the future (Lewin, 1943/1964c). Of all the potential causes of error identified by a person analyzing a misadventure, only those factors that actually influence the provider—be they past, present or future—drive the person on the path to error. The life-space of a care provider is illustrated in Fig. 13.1 as the disk behind the provider indicating that it is the driving force in his or her behavior.

Factors that fuel the engine of the life-space can be physiological in origin, such as hunger, the effects of a cold remedy, or aching legs due to varicose veins; psychological, as in concern about financial matters; and physical, such as difficult-to-use instruments. Influences in the life-space also may be immediate to the person, such as an argumentative colleague, or removed in time and space yet influencing the person, as in reimbursement policies that by not covering certain tests effectively restrict the information available about a patient's condition.

Factors external to the person are present in his or her life-space as their influences are experienced by the person. For example, laparoscopic instruments in

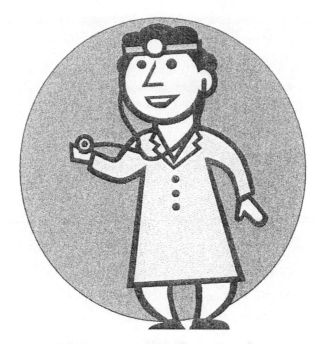

FIG. 13.1.   The life space of the care provider.

the operating room influence the surgeon's life-space when he or she anticipates or experiences problems using them. Otherwise, the mere existence of the instruments in the vicinity is not sufficient for them to influence the surgeon's life-space.

The waypoints or landmarks that define the path are events whose effect influences the care provider along the journey to error. Events such as a blow-out caused by the pothole of organizational factors when mandatory overtime for nurses was instituted affect the life-space of the care provider, which influences the determination of the path to error. Another person can observe factors in the context of care that appear to influence the care provider which indeed might be in his or her life-space; unless confirmed by the person observed, those factors can be misleading as in objective assessments.

The concept of life-space is useful in addressing a misadventure because its focus is on factors and events that are instrumental at the point of an error; the way points on the path to error. Although the analogy of the path to error conveys the importance of time in analyzing error, to be useful in identifying factors to be changed to reduce the likelihood of error, the consideration of the waypoints must be expanded. Addressing error as drama does that.

ERROR AS DRAMA

As Schliemann discovered the treasures of Troy by taking the writings of Homer literally and excavating the land accordingly, so might the analogy of staged drama assist the analysis of error by pursuing the double meaning, the *double entendre,* of words of the theater that are common to everyday parlance.

At least since the time of the Greeks, stories have been told, legends perpetrated, moral lessons taught, exploits heralded, and political and religious statements made through the medium of the theater. Shakespeare, the astute chronicler of human behavior, characterized the world and the human condition as theater— a characterization that indicates the value of the technique of expressing error as drama. Thus, an error is a dramatic performance. The structure of a performance is applied to the error context, and ultimately to selected inside stories.

Drama as an Analytical Aid

A performance is divided into Acts, which through a *double entendre* interpretation of an act as behavior, the Act of a drama is the incident in which the behavior, the error, occurred that precipitated the adverse outcome. As the Acts of a production may be divided into Scenes that portray changes in time and location, the analogy of error as an Act can force the consideration of Scenes and introduces the influence of changes in time and location on the conditions of the error. Conditions that occur prior to the error can set the stage or prime the context of care to increase the likelihood of error. Such preceding conditions have been referred to as *precursor events* that typically are identified as contributing to the error after an error has occurred. How much better for the prevention of errors it would be if the error-inducing properties of an event could be identified *prior* to it becoming a precursor.

To acknowledge that an error is related to conditions occurring prior in time and probably at a location other than that of the adverse outcome, that is, waypoints that occur early in the journey on the path to error, error is referred to as an episode rather than the mere error, which can imply the concept of a static error-as-a-photo. The Acts of a play, the Scenes, the stage directions, indeed all aspects of a performance including the actions and lines of the actor are scripted. The script is the dynamic representation of factors expressed in a systems approach to error (Bogner, 2000).

The Script of Error

The story of a performance exists in a script that becomes alive through the actors. The technique of considering error as drama provides the structure for analyzing error by reversing that process. That is, the story of error from life by the imposition of the structure of a dramatic play becomes a script of an error performance. As the script establishes the Acts and Scenes that define time and place, it defines the error and context being addressed. The script also defines the environment, the context of the scenery, lighting, and props for the performance. The systems in the artichoke model described in chapter 1 are manifest in the script. Each actor embodies the scripted characteristics, says the scripted lines, and follows the stage directions prescribed by the script that are unique to the specific role of the actor. The actor's performance is the behavior representing the perspective of the role.

Script as Perspective

The script for Actor A does not contain the lines for the characters of Actor B or Actor C or for any other actor in the scene. The role of an actor, or the perspective of the character of that actor, can only be determined through the script of the character role of the specific actor. In describing an error, Actor A can relate A's interpretation of the activity of Actor B or Actor C, but cannot relate B's interpretation of the activity of any actor. Thus, the consideration of error as drama underscores an important point in considering error: The perspective of the person involved in an error is unique to that person. The driving force for the actor in any role is the influence of the life-space of that actor incorporated into that role.

Performance in Time

A play involves the passage of time — if it did not, it would be merely a tableau. The script of a play divides the performance into Acts, the double entendre of which means performing an act, doing something such as the behavior of providing health care. Because behaviors occur over time, whether a brief or extended period, the Acts specified by the script establish time for the performance. Each Act indicates major changes in time, such as years, or changes in the seasons or in location. The script can specify Scenes within the Acts that indicate passage of time by changes in location as well as changes in the time of day, day of week, month of year, or year.

Script as Determiner

An individual actor is selected to perform a specific role. If, for some reason, that individual is unable to perform, another actor assumes the role. Although actors vary in their interpretation of a given role, the performance by different actors essentially is the same in terms of outcome of their performance because the performance is determined by the script. In health care misadventures, the script of context of care governs the performance of a care provider; that is, factors in the context contribute to, if not provoke, error. Performance in a specific context of care is similar for different individuals who fit the characteristics of the role, such as surgeons with comparable training. Thus, given that the scripted context of care determines the outcome of a performance, removing a provider who was involved in an error is not effective in reducing the likelihood of recurrence of the error. To effectively alter the performance outcome, the script must be changed.

INSIGHTS FROM THE INSIDE STORIES

To illustrate its usefulness in unraveling the web of factors that is the context of an error, the technique of error as drama is applied to aspects of two of the inside stories.

An Error Episode Drama in Five Acts

Although many factors that contributed to Sam Cohen's death were described in chapter 2, it would not be surprising if the attention of the reader were focused on Shirley Brown, the surgical intensive care nurse who transfused Mr. Cohen with incompatible blood and didn't recognize the early signs of a transfusion reaction. The drama technique forces the consideration of possible contributing factors. The application of the technique finds that to focus on Shirley Brown is to focus on an Act well into the drama.

Because drama unfolds over time, what preceded hanging the blood must be addressed. Laura Peterson, a blood bank technologist, released the blood for another patient as blood for Sam Cohen. Again, the preceding Act must be identified—the Act of assigning patient identifiers in the Emergency Room (ER). Yet again, the preceding Act must be considered—the Act of the accident with a flashback that Sam went running without any personal identification. This is Act 1, the first waypoint on the road to error that ultimately killed Sam Cohen.

The numbers of the Acts, the waypoints, occurred in reverse order of their presentation in the discussion, with the Act in which Shirley Brown hangs the blood being Act 4. The mere identification of that being Act 4 underscores the presence of precursor events; had these events not happened, the incident would not have occurred. It is to be noted that the Acts can have a number of Scenes which, although present in the story, are not included in this discussion for the sake of expediency. The value of differentiating the Scenes within an Act as well as the Acts is to identify strands in the tangle of the web of error so each can be addressed as appropriate.

The application of the error-as-drama technique should force the consideration of the final Act of what occurs after the error. That Act should have at least two Scenes—of the immediate actions and of the effect of those actions. Scene 1 of the final Act in the case of Sam Cohen shows Shirley Brown and Laura Peterson being allowed to resign rather than be dismissed. In Scene 2, the ER staff is assigning the same type of patient identifiers as the unidentified Sam Cohen received.

It may be noted that the backward chaining of Acts is similar to asking why for each act. The value of the drama technique is to probe for an Act, a dynamic behavior, rather than allowing a response of a static name of a category. Each Act can be analyzed for factors in the artichoke of the context of error that contributed to that behavior. For example, observations of the Blood Bank where Laura Peterson released a bag of blood for the wrong patient could find that the refrigerator for storing the blood had no sections to separate the blood by type, hence the bags of the types of blood could become intermingled and set the stage for an error.

An Error Episode Drama in Three Acts

Mrs. Bledsoe (chapter 12) took five 5 mg tablets when she was told by the nurse to take five, which the nurse intended to convey as the 5 mg of one tablet. This is Act 2 of the performance. Act 1 occurred when the prescription was written and filled with directions to "take 5 mg as directed." That created the precursor condition. With no directions as to how many tablets to take, Mrs. Bledsoe must remember what she is told in the physician's office or over the phone. She has no written directions to check.

The all-important final Act consists of the Scene of the typical reaction to Mrs. Bledsoe's error; she is scolded because she wasn't paying attention. The second Scene in the final Act finds prescriptions written for other patients and filled with the directions to "take 5 mg as directed." The nurse, however, is more explicit in her phoned instructions for dosage.

ALL THE WORLD'S A STAGE

The contribution of the discussion of the path to error and the technique of error as drama to address misadventures in health care, although far from being fully elaborated, has provided noteworthy insights for the analysis of error. Those insights are that it is critical to address time as a factor in error because error is not static; the journey on the road to error, that is the drama of error, occurs over time. A related insight is that conditions that lead to misadventures accumulate over time; events precede and set the stage for adverse outcomes. Precursor events are the culprits in error. If those conditions were rectified, the likelihood of error would decrease.

Although it is tempting to leave the policing of error-inducing situations to the patient safety community, the problem is too great for any community, no matter how well intentioned, to conquer. It is incumbent upon every concerned person to become active performers in addressing episodes of error by identifying precursor events and factors that contribute to error and to act to rectify them personally as appropriate. Mrs. Bledsoe can purchase labels, put specific instructions on a label and stick it on the pill bottle. When the instructions change, she can put a new label on the container.

For conditions that an individual can't correct, that person can notify the responsible party and follow up to be certain that the problem was corrected. If anyone at the hospital where Sam Cohen died had identified the initially assigned patient identifier as a significant precursor event, they could have contacted the hospital to change the way of assigning those identifiers. Shirley Brown, had she not been relieved of her duties, might have done that and prevented future misadventures. If, upon following up, one finds that nothing has been done and there is no intention to take action, then the individual should pursue having the problem addressed effectively by contacting a related professional organization or the media.

The emphasis of the reporting activities is on error and adverse outcomes— and well it should be. As is apparent in the inside stories that describe potential errors and incidents waiting to happen, the waypoints on the road to error, and the precursor events in the early Acts and Scenes of the drama of an error episode, it is important if not vital to reducing the likelihood of error that the conditions of those potential errors be identified and addressed. Aviation provides a poignant lesson to be learned. United Airlines cockpit crews knew a certain flight path approach to Dulles Airport from the west was dangerous and that it was an accident waiting to happen. Indeed, some pilots had experienced near accidents on that flight path; however, there was no existing mechanism for bringing the problem to the attention of pilots of other airlines or to those who could change the flight path. At 11:09 a.m. on Dec. 1, 1974, TWA Flight #514 crashed into the Blue Ridge Mountains, killing all 300 persons aboard (Reynard, Billings, Cheaney, & Hardy, 1986). Had the precursor conditions of the flight path and the lack of a means of getting information to pilots of other airlines been changed, the crash would not have occurred.

There are no dramatic disasters in health care such as plane crashes. Nonetheless, the lack of disaster is no excuse for inaction. The most conservative estimate of the number of people who die each year, not including those who require prolonged treatment and those who are injured, far exceeds the loss of life by transportation accidents. Reducing the likelihood of error in health care requires changing or removing error-provoking factors from the script of the context of care, not removing the care provider and introducing another into the same script.

Identifying factors that affect the provider in ways that contribute to error determines targets not only for remedial activity for health care organizations and topics for research or study by academic disciplines, but also—and perhaps more importantly—determines targets for device design changes by industry, and legislative changes by policy makers. Those policy changes should be directed not to the symptoms of the problem of misadventure in health care, that of errors, but to the legal, regulatory, and reimbursement sources of the problem.

REFERENCES

Bogner, M. S. (2000). A systems approach to medical error. In C. Vincent & B. De Mol (Eds.), *Safety in medicine* (pp. 83–101). Amsterdam: Pergamon.

Kelly, G. A. (1963). *A theory of personality: The psychology of personal constructs.* New York: Norton & Company.

Gaba, D. M. (1994). Human error in dynamic medical domains. In M. S. Bogner (Ed.), *Human error in medicine* (pp. 197–224). Mahwah, NJ: Lawrence Erlbaum Associates.

Gold, M. (1999). The making of a complete social scientist: A brief intellectual biography. In M. Gold (Ed.), *The complete social scientist: A Kurt Lewin Reader* (pp. 7–16). Washington, DC: American Psychological Association.

Kohn, L. T., & Corrigan, J. M. (Eds.). (1999). *To err is human: Building a safer health care system.* Washington, DC: National Academy Press.

Lewin, K. (1964a). Formalization and progress in psychology. In D. Cartwright (Ed.), *Field theory in social science* (pp. 1–30). New York: Harper & Row.

Lewin, K. (1964b). Field theory and learning. In D. Cartwright (Ed.), *Field theory in social science* (pp. 60–86). New York: Harper & Row.

Lewin, K. (1964c). Defining the "field at a given time." In D. Cartwright (Ed.), *Field theory in social science* (pp. 43–59). New York: Harper & Row.

Rasmussen, J. (1990). Human error and the problem of causality in analysis of accidents. *Philosophical Transactions of the Royal Society of London, B 327,* 449–462.

Reynard, W. C., Billings, C. E., Cheaney, E. S., & Hardy, R. (1986). *The development of the NASA aviation safety reporting system* (NASA Reference Publication 1114). Washington, DC: National Aeronautics and Space Administration.

Sjoerdsma, W. (1998). *Surgeons at work: Time and action analysis of the laparoscopic surgical process.* Doctoral dissertation, Delft Technical University, The Netherlands.

Traill, D. A. (1995). *Schliemann of Troy: Treasure and deceit.* New York: St. Martin's Griffin.

Author Index

Subject Index